T0226980

MRI of the Elbow and Wrist

Editor

KIMBERLY K. AMRAMI

MAGNETIC RESONANCE IMAGING CLINICS OF NORTH AMERICA

www.mri.theclinics.com

Consulting Editors
SURESH K. MUKHERJI
LYNNE S. STEINBACH

August 2015 • Volume 23 • Number 3

ELSEVIER

1600 John F. Kennedy Boulevard • Suite 1800 • Philadelphia, Pennsylvania, 19103-2899

http://www.mri.theclinics.com

MRI CLINICS OF NORTH AMERICA Volume 23, Number 3
August 2015 ISSN 1064-9689, ISBN 13: 978-0-323-39342-3

Editor: John Vassallo (j.vassallo@elsevier.com)
Developmental Editor: Meredith Clinton

© **2015 Elsevier Inc. All rights reserved.**

This periodical and the individual contributions contained in it are protected under copyright by Elsevier, and the following terms and conditions apply to their use:

Photocopying

Single photocopies of single articles may be made for personal use as allowed by national copyright laws. Permission of the Publisher and payment of a fee is required for all other photocopying, including multiple or systematic copying, copying for advertising or promotional purposes, resale, and all forms of document delivery. Special rates are available for educational institutions that wish to make photocopies for non-profit educational classroom use. For information on how to seek permission visit www.elsevier.com/permissions or call: (+44) 1865 843830 (UK)/ (+1) 215 239 3804 (USA).

Derivative Works

Subscribers may reproduce tables of contents or prepare lists of articles including abstracts for internal circulation within their institutions. Permission of the Publisher is required for resale or distribution outside the institution. Permission of the Publisher is required for all other derivative works, including compilations and translations (please consult www.elsevier.com/permissions).

Electronic Storage or Usage

Permission of the Publisher is required to store or use electronically any material contained in this periodical, including any article or part of an article (please consult www.elsevier.com/permissions). Except as outlined above, no part of this publication may be reproduced, stored in a retrieval system or transmitted in any form or by any means, electronic, mechanical, photocopying, recording or otherwise, without prior written permission of the Publisher.

Notice

No responsibility is assumed by the Publisher for any injury and/or damage to persons or property as a matter of products liability, negligence or otherwise, or from any use or operation of any methods, products, instructions or ideas contained in the material herein. Because of rapid advances in the medical sciences, in particular, independent verification of diagnoses and drug dosages should be made.

Although all advertising material is expected to conform to ethical (medical) standards, inclusion in this publication does not constitute a guarantee or endorsement of the quality or value of such product or of the claims made of it by its manufacturer.

Magnetic Resonance Imaging Clinics of North America (ISSN 1064-9689) is published quarterly by Elsevier Inc., 360 Park Avenue South, New York, NY 10010-1710. Months of issue are February, May, August, and November. Business and Editorial Offices: 1600 John F. Kennedy Blvd., Ste. 1800, Philadelphia, PA 19103-2899. Customer Service Office: 3251 Riverport Lane, Maryland Heights, MO 63043. Periodicals postage paid at New York, NY and additional mailing offices. Subscription prices are $375.00 per year (domestic individuals), $581.00 per year (domestic institutions), $190.00 per year (domestic students/residents), $420.00 per year (Canadian individuals), $755.00 per year (Canadian institutions), $545.00 per year (international individuals), $755.00 per year (international institutions), and $275.00 per year (international and Canadian students/residents). International air speed delivery is included in all *Clinics* subscription prices. All prices are subject to change without notice. **POSTMASTER:** Send address changes to *Magnetic Resonance Imaging Clinics*, Elsevier Health Sciences Division, Subscription Customer Service, 3251 Riverport Lane, Maryland Heights, MO 63043. Customer Service (orders, claims, online, change of address): Elsevier Health Sciences Division, Subscription **Customer Service, 3251 Riverport Lane, Maryland Heights, MO 63043. Tel:1-800-654-2452 (U.S. and Canada); 314-447-8871 (outside U.S. and Canada). Fax: 314-447-8029. E-mail: journalscustomer service-usa@elsevier.com (for print support); journalsonlinesupport-usa@elsevier.com (for online support).**

Reprints. For copies of 100 or more of articles in this publication, please contact the Commercial Reprints Department, Elsevier Inc., 360 Park Avenue South, New York, NY 10010-1710. Tel.: 212-633-3874; Fax: 212-633-3820; E-mail: reprints@elsevier.com.

Magnetic Resonance Imaging Clinics of North America is covered in the *RSNA Index of Imaging Literature, MEDLINE/PubMed (Index Medicus),* and *EMBASE/Excerpta Medica.*

Contributors

CONSULTING EDITORS

SURESH K. MUKHERJI, MD, MBA, FACR
Professor and Chairman; W.F. Patenge
Endowed Chair, Department of Radiology,
Michigan State University, East Lansing,
Michigan

LYNNE S. STEINBACH, MD, FACR
Professor of Radiology and Orthopaedic
Surgery, Department of Radiology and
Biomedical Imaging, University of California
San Francisco, San Francisco, California

EDITOR

KIMBERLY K. AMRAMI, MD
Professor of Radiology; Consultant in
Radiology and Neurologic Surgery; Chair,
Division of Musculoskeletal Radiology, Mayo
Clinic, Rochester, Minnesota

AUTHORS

TOSHI ABE, MD, PhD
Department of Radiology, Kurume University
School of Medicine, Kurume, Fukuoka, Japan

LAURA W. BANCROFT, MD
Department of Radiology, Florida Hospital;
Clinical Professor, University of Central Florida
College of Medicine, Orlando, Florida

PETER BANNAS, MD
Department of Radiology, University of
Wisconsin-Madison, Madison, Wisconsin;
Department of Radiology, University Hospital
Hamburg-Eppendorf, Hamburg, Germany

DANIELA BINAGHI, MD
Radiology Department, Favaloro University,
Favaloro Foundation, Buenos Aires,
Argentina

MICHAEL E. CODY, MD
Department of Radiology, Brigham and
Women's Hospital, Boston, Massachusetts

TRISTAN DE MOOIJ, MD
Departments of Neurologic Surgery and
Orthopedic Surgery, Mayo Clinic, Rochester,
Minnesota

ERIC C. EHMAN, MD
Department of Radiology and Biomedical
Imaging, University of California, San
Francisco, San Francisco, California

JOEL P. FELMLEE, PhD
Department of Radiology, Mayo Clinic,
Rochester, Minnesota

CHRISTOPHER J. FRANÇOIS, MD
Department of Radiology, University of
Wisconsin-Madison, Madison, Wisconsin

MATTHEW A. FRICK, MD
Department of Radiology, Mayo Clinic,
Rochester, Minnesota

GARRY E. GOLD, MD
Departments of Radiology, Bioengineering,
and Orthopaedic Surgery, Stanford University,
Stanford, California

BENJAMIN MATTHEW HOWE, MD
Department of Radiology, Mayo Clinic,
Rochester, Minnesota

DUSTIN JOHNSON, MD
Department of Radiology, Stanford University,
Stanford, California

SANJEEV KAKAR, MD, MRCS
Associate Professor, Department of Orthopedic Surgery, Mayo Clinic, Rochester, Minnesota

GARY M. LiMARZI, MD
PGY-3 Radiology Resident, Florida Hospital Diagnostic Radiology Residency Program, Department of Radiology, Florida Hospital, Instructor, University of Central Florida College of Medicine, Orlando, Florida

NAVEEN S. MURTHY, MD
Associate Professor, Division of Musculoskeletal Radiology, Department of Radiology, Mayo Clinic, Rochester, Minnesota

SHUJI NAGATA, MD, PhD
Department of Radiology, Kurume University School of Medicine, Kurume, Fukuoka, Japan

DAVID T. NAKAMURA, MD
Department of Radiology, UC Davis Medical Center, Sacramento, California

HIROSHI NISHIMURA, MD, PhD
Department of Radiology, Saiseikai Futsukaichi Hospital, Chikushino, Fukuoka, Japan

M. CODY O'DELL, MD
PGY-4 Radiology Resident, Florida Hospital Diagnostic Radiology Residency Program, Department of Radiology, Florida Hospital, Instructor, University of Central Florida College of Medicine, Orlando, Florida

CHRISTOPHER PETTIS, MD
Department of Radiology, Florida Hospital; Clinical Assistant Professor, University of Central Florida College of Medicine, Orlando, Florida

SCOTT B. REEDER, MD, PhD
Departments of Radiology, Biomedical Engineering, Medical Physics, Medicine, and Emergency Medicine, University of Wisconsin-Madison, Madison, Wisconsin

SCOTT RIESTER, MD
Department of Orthopedic Surgery, Mayo Clinic, Rochester, Minnesota

GEOFFREY RILEY, MD
Department of Radiology, Stanford University, Stanford, California

MICHAEL D. RINGLER, MD
Assistant Professor, Division of Musculoskeletal Radiology, Department of Radiology, Mayo Clinic, Rochester, Minnesota

KURT SCHERER, MD
Department of Radiology, Florida Hospital; Clinical Assistant Professor, University of Central Florida College of Medicine, Orlando, Florida

LAUREN SHAPIRO, MD
Department of Radiology, Stanford University, Stanford, California

KIRSTIN M. SMALL, MD
Department of Radiology, Brigham and Women's Hospital, Boston, Massachusetts

ROBERT J. SPINNER, MD
Department of Neurologic Surgery, Mayo Clinic, Rochester, Minnesota

KATHRYN J. STEVENS, MD
Departments of Radiology and Orthopaedic Surgery, Stanford University, Stanford, California

CHRISTOPHER W. WASYLIW, MD
Department of Radiology, Florida Hospital; Clinical Assistant Professor, University of Central Florida College of Medicine, Orlando, Florida

HIROSHI YOSHIOKA, MD, PhD
Department of Radiological Sciences, UC Irvine Medical Center; Department of Radiology, University of California, Orange, California

Contents

Wrist and elbow MR imaging technology is advancing at a dramatic rate. Wrist and elbow MR imaging is performed at medium and higher field strengths with more specialized surface coils and more variable pulse sequences and postprocessing techniques. High field imaging and improved coils lead to an increased signal-to-noise ratio and increased variety of soft tissue contrast options. Three-dimensional imaging is improving in terms of usability and artifacts. Some of these advances have challenges in wrist and elbow imaging, such as postoperative patient imaging, cartilage mapping, and molecular imaging. This review considers technical advances in hardware and software and their clinical applications.

This article discusses the normal anatomy and pathologic appearances of the intrinsic and extrinsic wrist ligaments using MR Imaging. Technological advances in surface coil design and higher magnetic field strengths have improved radiologists' ability to consistently visualize these small ligaments in their entirety. Wrist ligament anatomy, in the context of proper physiologic function, is emphasized, including common normal variants, and their appearances on MR imaging. The spectrum of disorders, incorporating overlapping appearances of senescent degenerative changes, and destabilizing ligament tears, is outlined. The diagnostic performance of MR imaging to date for various ligament abnormalities is discussed, along with significant limitations.

MR imaging has emerged as the mainstay in imaging internal derangement of the soft tissues of the musculoskeletal system largely because of superior contrast resolution. The complex geometry and diminutive size of the triangular fibrocartilage complex (TFCC) and its constituent structures can make optimal imaging of the TFCC challenging; therefore, production of clinically useful images requires careful optimization of image acquisition parameters. This article provides a foundation for advanced TFCC imaging including factors to optimize magnetic resonance images, arthrography, detailed anatomy, and classification of injury. In addition, clinical presentations and treatments for TFCC injury are briefly considered.

> Certain soft-tissue tumors seem to be specific to the upper extremity; most are benign. Knowledge of key magnetic resonance features, with clinical history and epidemiologic knowledge, can assist the radiologist in establishing optimal diagnosis. Indeterminate lesions require biopsy to exclude malignancy.

> The peripheral nervous system is susceptible to a diverse array of pathologic insults. The pathology may be intrinsic to the nerves themselves, either primarily arising within the nerve(s) or direct involvement of the nerve(s) secondary to a systemic process, or external to the nerve(s) proper but affecting them extrinsically via mass effect, such as entrapment neuropathies. The soft tissue contrast and resolution inherent to high-quality MR imaging allows for outstanding visualization of the peripheral nervous system and surrounding structures. This review focuses on the use of MR imaging in the diagnosis and management of peripheral nerve disorders of the upper extremity.

> The magnetic resonance angiography (MRA) toolbox includes a wide array of versatile methods for diagnosis and therapy planning in patients with a variety of upper extremity vascular pathologies. MRA can provide excellent image quality with high spatial and high temporal resolution without the disadvantages of ionizing radiation, iodinated contrast, and operator dependency. Contrast-enhanced techniques are preferred for their robustness, image quality, and shorter scan times. This article provides an overview of the available MRA techniques and a description of the clinical entities that are well suited for evaluation with contrast-enhanced MRA.

> The introduction of 3-T MR imaging scanners as well as dedicated wrist coils has allowed for scanning of the unique anatomic structures within the hand with increasing accuracy. In this article, the authors discuss common hand conditions, focusing on imaging findings and the utility of MR imaging as it pertains to hand surgery. The authors examine its role in the treatment of hand deep-space infections, scaphoid fractures, scapholunate ligament injuries, thumb ulnar collateral ligament injuries, and ulnar-sided wrist pain.

MAGNETIC RESONANCE IMAGING CLINICS OF NORTH AMERICA

RELATED INTEREST

VISIT THE CLINICS ONLINE!
Access your subscription at:
www.theclinics.com

PROGRAM OBJECTIVE

The goal of *Magnetic Resonance Imaging Clinics of North America* is to keep practicing physicians up to date with current clinical practice by providing timely articles reviewing the state of the art in patient care.

TARGET AUDIENCE

All practicing physicians and healthcare professionals who provide patient care utilizing findings from Magnetic Resonance Imaging.

LEARNING OBJECTIVES

Upon completion of this activity, participants will be able to:
1. Recognize the applications of MR imaging in upper extremity abnormalities such as fractures and soft tissue tumors.
2. Discuss methods of MR imaging of nerves, ligaments, and soft tissue in the upper extremity.
3. Review techniques in imaging the joints of the wrist and elbow.

ACCREDITATION

The Elsevier Office of Continuing Medical Education (EOCME) is accredited by the Accreditation Council for Continuing Medical Education (ACCME) to provide continuing medical education for physicians.

The EOCME designates this enduring material for a maximum of 15 *AMA PRA Category 1 Credit*(s)™. Physicians should claim only the credit commensurate with the extent of their participation in the activity.

All other health care professionals requesting continuing education credit for this enduring material will be issued a certificate of participation.

DISCLOSURE OF CONFLICTS OF INTEREST

The EOCME assesses conflict of interest with its instructors, faculty, planners, and other individuals who are in a position to control the content of CME activities. All relevant conflicts of interest that are identified are thoroughly vetted by EOCME for fair balance, scientific objectivity, and patient care recommendations. EOCME is committed to providing its learners with CME activities that promote improvements or quality in healthcare and not a specific proprietary business or a commercial interest.

The planning committee, staff, authors and editors listed below have identified no financial relationships or relationships to products or devices they or their spouse/life partner have with commercial interest related to the content of this CME activity:

Toshi Abe, MD, PhD; Kimberly K. Amrami, MD; Laura W. Bancroft, MD; Peter Bannas, MD; Daniela Binaghi, MD; Michael E. Cody, MD; Tristan de Mooij, MD; Eric C. Ehman, MD; Joel P. Felmlee, PhD; Anjali Fortna; Christopher J. François, MD; Matthew A. Frick, MD; Benjamin Matthew Howe, MD; Dustin Johnson, MD; Gary M. LiMarzi, MD; Suresh K. Mukherji, MD, MBA, FACR; Naveen S. Murthy, MD; Shuji Nagata, MD, PhD; David T. Nakamura, MD; Hiroshi Nishimura, MD, PhD; M. Cody O'Dell, MD; Christopher Pettis, MD; Scott B. Reeder, MD, PhD; Scott Riester, MD; Geoffrey Riley, MD; Michael D. Ringler, MD; Kurt Scherer, MD; Lauren Shapiro, MD; Kirstin M. Small, MD; Lynne S. Steinbach, MD, FACR; Kathryn J. Stevens, MD; Karthikeyan Subramaniam; Megan Suermann; John Vassallo; Christopher W. Wasyliw, MD; Hiroshi Yoshioka, MD, PhD.

The planning committee, staff, authors and editors listed below have identified financial relationships or relationships to products or devices they or their spouse/life partner have with commercial interest related to the content of this CME activity:

Garry E. Gold, MD is a consultant/advisor for Olea Medical and Boston Scientific Corporation, and has research support from GE Healthcare, a subsidiary of General Electric Company.

Sanjeev Kakar, MD, MRCS is a consultant/advisor for Arthrex, Inc. and Skeletal Dynamics LLC, and has research support from Arthrex, Inc.

Robert J. Spinner, MD is a consultant/advisor for Mayo Clinic Ventures, part of the Mayo Foundation for Medical Education and Research.

UNAPPROVED/OFF-LABEL USE DISCLOSURE

The EOCME requires CME faculty to disclose to the participants:
1. When products or procedures being discussed are off-label, unlabelled, experimental, and/or investigational (not US Food and Drug Administration (FDA) approved; and
2. Any limitations on the information presented, such as data that are preliminary or that represent ongoing research, interim analyses, and/or unsupported opinions. Faculty may discuss information about pharmaceutical agents that is outside of FDA-approved labelling. This information is intended solely for CME and is not intended to promote off-label use of these medications. If you have any questions, contact the medical affairs department of the manufacturer for the most recent prescribing information.

TO ENROLL

To enroll in the *Magnetic Resonance Imaging Clinics of North America* Continuing Medical Education program, call customer service at 1-800-654-2452 or sign up online at http://www.theclinics.com/home/cme. The CME program is available to subscribers for an additional annual fee of USD 250.

METHOD OF PARTICIPATION
In order to claim credit, participants must complete the following:
1. Complete enrolment as indicated above.
2. Read the activity.
3. Complete the CME Test and Evaluation. Participants must achieve a score of 70% on the test. All CME Tests and Evaluations must be completed online.

CME INQUIRIES/SPECIAL NEEDS
For all CME inquiries or special needs, please contact elsevierCME@elsevier.com.

Foreword
MR Imaging of the Elbow and Wrist

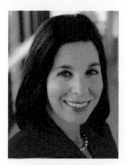

Lynne S. Steinbach, MD, FACR
Consulting Editor

I am pleased to introduce this issue of *Magnetic Resonance Imaging Clinics of North America* that focuses on the elbow and wrist. It is refreshing to have some updated information on this complex subject. These joints are rather challenging to evaluate and understand, and there have been many technological developments in the last few years that have improved their imaging.

Dr Kimberly Amrami, Professor of Radiology at the Mayo Clinic, Rochester, is spearheading this project as guest editor. Dr Amrami has an excellent knowledge of the subject, including the anatomy, pathology, and technical challenges and details.

A cadre of distinguished radiologists and orthopedic surgeons discusses various important topics regarding MR imaging of the elbow and wrist. Authors include physicians from world-renowned medical centers, including Mayo Clinic, Stanford, Florida Hospital, University of California San Francisco, University of Wisconsin, Brigham and Women's, University of California Irvine, Favaloro University in Buenos Aires, and Kurume University in Japan.

The content of this issue is timely. New sequences that reduce metal artifact and other techniques, such as isotropic imaging, uTE imaging, T2- and T1-rho mapping, are discussed. Techniques such as MR arthrography, MR angiography, and MR neurography are covered in different articles. Anatomy and pathology in the elbow are succinctly presented. Separate reviews of wrist ligaments, the triangular fibrocartilage, proximal and distal radioulnar joints, carpal fractures, and soft tissue tumors of the upper extremity provide the detail that is needed for today's imager. In addition, there is a valuable synopsis regarding the relevance of MR imaging to hand surgeons.

Thank you, Dr Amrami and your team of authors, for your hard work to create this exciting and valuable collection of information on these various important topics in the area of MR imaging of the elbow and wrist.

Lynne S. Steinbach, MD, FACR
Department of Radiology and Biomedical Imaging
University of California San Francisco
505 Parnassus
San Francisco, CA 94143-0628, USA

E-mail address:
lynne.steinbach@ucsf.edu

Magn Reson Imaging Clin N Am 23 (2015) xi
http://dx.doi.org/10.1016/j.mric.2015.05.002
1064-9689/15/$ – see front matter © 2015 Published by Elsevier Inc.

Preface
MR Imaging of the Wrist and Elbow

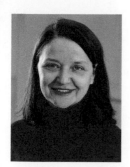

Kimberly K. Amrami, MD
Editor

MR imaging has become an important tool in the evaluation of the wrist and elbow. Advances in MR imaging, including the use of 3T and dedicated receiver coils for routine imaging, have made high-resolution clinical imaging routine and reproducible. Structures such as nerves and tiny ligaments once impossible to visualize are now seen clearly and in detail. Because of this, clinical expectations have risen, and an understanding of the anatomy and pathologic processes affecting these complicated joints has become more and more important. The talented authors in this issue have provided articles covering the full gamut of MR imaging of the wrist and elbow, including advanced imaging techniques, anatomy, and a review of common and less common conditions affecting the upper extremity. In this issue, you will find articles that will take you through the full range of information needed to perform, understand, and interpret MR imaging of the wrist and elbow. You will also gain an understanding of new and evolving developments and technologies that continue to push the boundaries of the newest and more advanced MR techniques available for the wrist and elbow, specifically, including angiography, neurography, arthrography, and dynamic 4D kinematic imaging.

This issue on MR of the Wrist and Elbow takes a fresh look at the basics of imaging the ligaments, nerves, and vessels of the joints of the upper extremity as well as discusses more esoteric topics as the biomechanics of the elbow and wrist joints as it relates to imaging, both static and dynamic.

Tumors, common and rare, and neurogenic and vascular conditions are discussed in detail. The issue is rounded out with an article by Drs de Mooij, Riester, and Kakar on the relevance of MR imaging of the wrist and elbow from a surgeon's perspective, reminding us that as radiologists we do not work in a vacuum but rather contribute a critical element to patient care with high-quality, tailored exams that are then interpreted based on deep understanding of the clinical problems to be addressed. This collaboration of clinicians and radiologists has driven much of the evolution and progress of MR imaging in this area; it continues to drive innovation and development of new technologies, such as dynamic and kinematic imaging, to address complex clinical problems, such as carpal instability.

This expert team of authors has created a complete and expert set of works, and I am truly grateful for their efforts and contributions. I believe that this issue will serve as a source of information for radiologists and clinicians alike and that all readers, from trainees to the most expert subspecialists, will find something to learn here.

Kimberly K. Amrami, MD
Department of Radiology
Mayo Clinic
200 1st Street Southwest
Rochester, MN 55905, USA

E-mail address:
amrami.kimberly@mayo.edu

Magn Reson Imaging Clin N Am 23 (2015) xiii
http://dx.doi.org/10.1016/j.mric.2015.05.001
1064-9689/15/$ – see front matter © 2015 Published by Elsevier Inc.

Approach to MR Imaging of the Elbow and Wrist
Technical Aspects and Innovation

Dustin Johnson, MD[a], Kathryn J. Stevens, MD[a,b],
Geoffrey Riley, MD[a], Lauren Shapiro, MD[a],
Hiroshi Yoshioka, MD, PhD[c], Garry E. Gold, MD[a,b,d],*

KEYWORDS

- MR imaging • Wrist • Elbow • High field imaging • Phased array coils • Metallic implants
- Isotropic imaging • Cartilage mapping

KEY POINTS

- Positioning of the subject near isocenter of the scanner results in the best image quality in terms of artifacts and fat suppression.
- High field imaging (>1.5 T) with multichannel phased array coils results in the best anatomic and contrast resolution.
- New methods for motion compensation, imaging around metal, and evaluation of cartilage are becoming more widely available.

INTRODUCTION

Since its introduction in the 1970s, MR imaging has revolutionized the diagnosis and treatment of musculoskeletal disorders. MR imaging has proven to be a valuable imaging tool in almost every joint in the body as a result of its ability to assess a wide range of anatomy and pathologies, ranging from ligamentous injuries to articular cartilage lesions.[1–3] With its multiplanar capabilities and excellent soft tissue contrast, MR imaging has established itself as one of the most promising modalities for noninvasive evaluation of the musculoskeletal system.[4,5]

The wrist and elbow are now evaluated commonly with MR imaging. Because of the mobility and location of the wrist and elbow, both can be imaged in a variety of positions using different types of coils. These locations have trade-offs in terms of patient motion and image artifacts. Most issues with imaging of these joints have been mitigated with technical advances in scanner hardware and software. Along with these improvements in technology, however, come various new technical challenges that need to be considered and understood.

LOW FIELD IMAGING

MR imaging at field strengths below 1.5 T is becoming less common, but is still frequently used for wrist and elbow imaging. Dedicated low field strength scanners such as the Artoscan (Esaote, Inc, Indianapolis, IN, USA) are able to produce intermediate quality images of these joints, and can be more comfortable for the patient. In addition, specialized coils can produce high-resolution images, despite the relatively low field strength (Fig. 1). Low field MR imaging of the wrist is common

The authors, and research, in this article are supported by NIH EB002524, NIH K24062068, GE Healthcare, Wrist and Elbow Musculoskeletal MRI – Technical Considerations.

[a] Department of Radiology, Stanford University, Stanford, CA, USA; [b] Department of Orthopaedic Surgery, Stanford University, Stanford, CA, USA; [c] Department of Radiology, University of California, Irvine, CA, USA; [d] Department of Bioengineering, Stanford University, Stanford, CA, USA
* Corresponding author. Department of Radiology, 1201 Welch Road, P263, Stanford, CA 94305.
E-mail address: gold@stanford.edu

1064-9689/15/$ – see front matter © 2015 Elsevier Inc. All rights reserved.

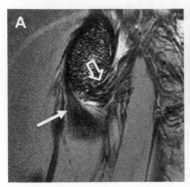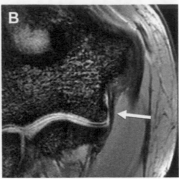

Fig. 1. Sagittal (A) and coronal (B) T2* images of the elbow obtained on a 1.5 T scanner using a 2-inch microscopy coil demonstrating the anterior (arrow) and posterior bands (open arrow) of the medial collateral ligament.

in the evaluation of rheumatoid arthritis[6,7] and is useful in scoring bony erosions and synovitis. It has also been demonstrated to be useful after wrist trauma.[8] Examination of the elbow with low field systems is less common than the wrist.

HIGH FIELD IMAGING

MR imaging of the wrist and elbow is now commonly performed at intermediate field strengths of 1.5 T or higher. Imaging at 3.0 T has become increasingly common for clinical evaluation, and even higher field systems (7.0 T) are being evaluated in the research realm.[9] Although initially used for neurologic imaging, numerous studies have confirmed the benefits and abilities of higher field systems in musculoskeletal imaging.[10–12] In particular, the development of dedicated coils has increased the utility of high field imaging. The most valuable benefit is an improved signal-to-noise ratio (SNR), which can result in increased image resolution (Fig. 2). Additionally, increased SNR affords the opportunity to shorten the examination time. However, with the increase in field strength to 3.0 T or higher, numerous technical factors must be considered to optimize its intrinsically superior imaging capabilities.

Although one would assume that doubling the field strength from 1.5 to 3.0 T should result in double the intrinsic SNR, it actually results in slightly less than a 2-fold increase because of changes in T1 relaxation times and complexities of coils at higher field strengths. Research measuring changes in relaxation times have shown that T1 relaxation times must be increased by 14% to 20% when moving from 1.5 to 3.0 T.[11] Increased off-resonance effects may result in higher receiver bandwidth for some sequences, which in turn, reduces SNR.

There are several technical considerations that must be addressed to take full advantage of 3.0 T and higher field imaging systems. The most prominent issues include chemical shift, fat saturation, and radiofrequency (RF) power deposition. Chemical shift displacement artifact doubles in the frequency encoding direction when moving from 1.5 to 3.0 T. Doubling the receiver bandwidth is one way to resolve this issue. Doubling the bandwidth not only corrects the chemical shift artifact, but may also allow for an increase in the number of slices acquired, decrease metal artifacts, shorten echo times, and reduce echo spacing. On the other hand, doubling the bandwidth decreases the SNR by a factor of $\sqrt{2}$, because the overall readout window length is shorter.

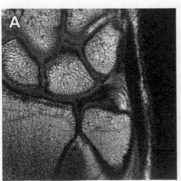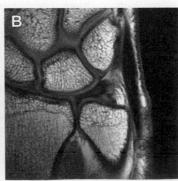

Fig. 2. Coronal T1 images of the triangular fibrocartilage of the wrist utilizing a microscopy coil demonstrating low signal-to-noise ratio (SNR) on image (A), and improved SNR and image quality on image (B), as can be seen with increasing magnetic field strength.

The doubled chemical shift difference between the fat and water resonance at 3.0 and 1.5 T makes fat saturation much easier. The peaks are twice as far apart with a chemical shift of 440 Hz, meaning that the lengths of the fat saturation pulses can be shortened from about 16 to 8 msec.[13] An advantage of this is the ability to acquire more slices at a given repetition time, bandwidth, and slice thickness.

RF power deposition is a third technical issue, especially in fast or turbo spin-echo sequences used in musculoskeletal imaging. RF power is proportional to the square of the field strength; therefore, it will quadruple when field strength is doubled from 1.5 to 3.0 T.[14,15] Although the overall deposition depends on the number of RF pulses and amplitude, using rapid imaging sequences with lower flip angles may minimize the deposition. When examining small volumes and using transmit receive coils, this complication should be diminished, because the RF power that is deposited is a function of the tissue volume excited.[15] However, many dedicated wrist and surface coils use the body coil to transmit RF energy and can result in high specific absorption rate (SAR).

It is more advantageous to use a localized transmit/receive RF coil than a body coil transmit; however, if a body coil transmit is used, shortening the examination time or lowering the refocusing pulses would help to limit SAR. The US Food and Drug Administration limitation for the whole body over a 15-minute period in all patients is 4 W/kg and for extremities over a period of 5 minutes the local SAR limit is 12 W/kg.[16,17]

The use of 7.0 T to image the musculoskeletal system is still in the early stages, and there are many technical problems, including SAR, chemical shift, and B1 homogeneity.[9,18,19] Routine imaging at 7.0 T could provide higher SNR, higher resolution, or more rapid imaging. Multichannel coils with parallel transmission capability are under development, which promise to improve image quality and lower SAR.

PHASED ARRAY COILS/PARALLEL IMAGING

Higher field strength MR imaging systems are being developed to increase SNR and improve resolution. However, tissue/field interactions often develop owing to a higher precession frequency and shorter wavelength, making it difficult to acquire high-quality images. Phased array coil technology was developed originally to improve the signal intensity uniformity of MR images obtained using surface coils and high field imaging, while preserving the inherent SNR gain. New methods for encoding the MR imaging signal are being adopted that fall under the generic name of "parallel imaging." Parallel imaging methods exploit the spatially varying sensitivity profiles of the surface coil elements within the array to extend the imaging field of view without adding additional scan time. This strategy allows a net reduction in the amount of time required to obtain the MR image up to a factor related to the number of independent coil channels within the array. Multiple channels are required to process the data independently, and in principle, an 8-channel coil would be able to image 8 times as fast, assuming an ideal geometry. However, practical considerations limit image acceleration to values below the theoretic maximum.

The clinical impact of parallel imaging is considerable for the higher field imaging of the wrist and elbow at 3.0 T. The use of parallel imaging technology can not only reduce scan time and the number of RF pulses required to form an image, but can also be used to shorten the echo time, which proves to be a significant improvement for musculoskeletal imaging. This will be important in limiting the total RF power to regulatory guidelines, particularly for wrist and elbow imaging with body coil transmit at 3.0 T. When parallel imaging is used, image uniformity and SNR are both compromised because scan times are reduced. Innovative phased array coil designs with up to 32 or more channels have been developed to accommodate parallel imaging methods at higher magnetic fields. The newest MR imaging systems are being offered with receiver system capacity for a highly scalable number of individual RF channels. The maximum number of RF channels that can practically be incorporated into the design of clinical MR imaging systems is controversial.

POSITIONING AND FAT SUPPRESSION

Ideally, the body part of interest is placed at the isocenter of the scanner, where magnetic field homogeneity and gradient uniformity are best. However, this can be challenging for wrist and elbow imaging. Placing the wrist or elbow at isocenter usually requires prone positioning with the arm of interest over the subjects head, the so-called "superman" position. This places the anatomy of interest in the best location for imaging, but can be uncomfortable and difficult to maintain for long periods of time, and therefore prone to motion artifact (Fig. 3A). Motion artifact can be improved by adding motion-insensitive sequences, such as propeller (see Fig. 3B), to the protocol.[20]

Modern phased-array multichannel coils allow placement of the wrist or elbow by the side of the patient in a supine position, which is more comfortable and less prone to motion. However,

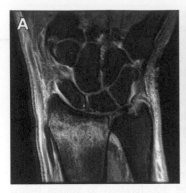

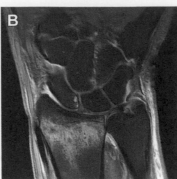

Fig. 3. (A) Coronal PD FS of the wrist showing mild motion artifact, which improves using a motion-insensitive sequence - Coronal PD FS Propeller (B).

this places the anatomy far from the isocenter, and achieving high-quality imaging with fat suppression can be difficult (**Fig. 4**A). Use of manual shimming and manual prescan to set the center frequency can often correct this problem (see **Fig. 4**B). Use of short Tau inversion recovery for fat suppression or methods of fat/water separation such as Iterative Decomposition of water and fat with Echo Asymmetry and Least-squares estimation (IDEAL) can also be helpful to obtain quality fat suppressed or fat–water separated images in areas of poor magnetic field homogeneiety.[21,22]

DIRECT AND INDIRECT MAGNETIC RESONANCE ARTHROGRAPHY

MR arthrography is an important alternative to conventional MR imaging of the wrist and elbow, particularly in cases where detailed evaluation of cartilage or ligaments is vital. Direct MR arthrography distends the joint compartment, allowing for better delineation and visualization between tissues. It also allows for detection of abnormal communication between joint compartments and between extraarticular soft tissues and joint compartments. The drawbacks of direct MR arthrography are that it is invasive, thereby introducing the

potential for infection, and exposes the patient to x-rays for procedure guidance.

Indirect MR arthrography is useful in joints that have less capacity for distension, and is less invasive than direct MR arthrography. A disadvantage of indirect MR arthrography is that contrast will be present in all components of the joint, preventing visualization of abnormal communication between joint compartments. In addition, the level of joint enhancement depends on joint volume, intraarticular pressure, blood concentration of contrast, inflammation and permeability, synovial area, and time delay after contrast injection.[23,24] Despite the drawbacks of both direct and indirect MR arthrography, these techniques have proven useful in the evaluation of most joints including the elbow and wrist.[25–27]

3.0 T MR IMAGING PROTOCOLS

Example 3T imaging protocols are included for the wrist (**Fig. 5, Table 1**) and the elbow (**Fig. 6, Table 2**). These protocols are relatively long in total scan time by modern standards, but include good coverage of the anatomy and high SNR and resolution. The important principle is to cover the joint in multiple planes and with multiple

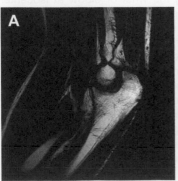

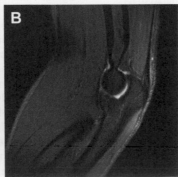

Fig. 4. Sagittal T2-weighted, fat-suppressed images of the elbow in a patient with acute trauma. Owing to the patient's trauma, the elbow was positioned near the side of the patient. (A) Initial T2-weighted image with failure of fat saturation owing to off resonance. (B) Improved fat saturation after manual shim and adjustment of center frequency.

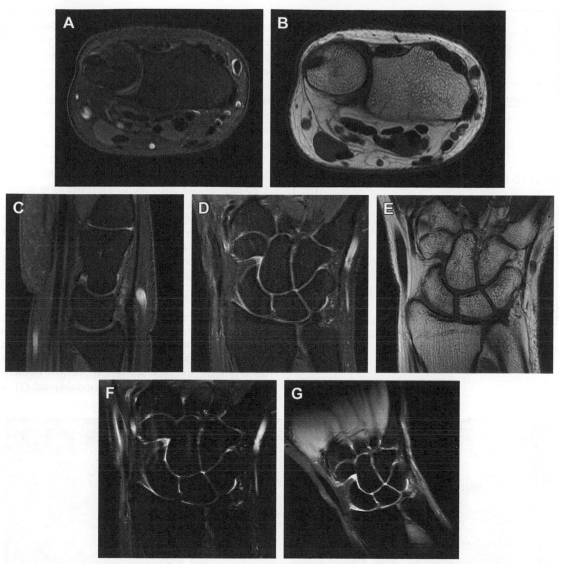

Fig. 5. Images from the 3T wrist protocol shown in **Table 2**, acquired in a patient with the 8-channel phased-array wrist coil. (*A*) Axial proton-density weighted (PD) with fat saturation (FS). (*B*) Axial T1-weighted image. (*C*) Sagittal PD FS image. (*D*) Coronal PD FS image. (*E*) Coronal T1-weighted image. (*F*) Coronal T2-weighted image. (*G*) Coronal Cube Flex image.

different tissue contrasts. Coronal images of the wrist are obtained by acquiring oblique slices oriented parallel to the ulnar and radial styloids (**Fig. 7**). Coronal images of the elbow are prescribed in plane with a line drawn along the anterior margin of the humerus at the level of the medial and lateral condyles (**Fig. 8**).

ISOTROPIC IMAGING

MR imaging of the musculoskeletal system is conventionally performed with 2-dimensional (2D) multislice acquisitions. Turbo spin-echo or fast spin-echo (FSE) acquisitions are used commonly,

because they provide excellent visualization of anatomy and pathology, including meniscal tears,[28,29] ligamentous injury,[30] and cartilage damage.[31] The drawback of 2D-FSE is that the voxels obtained are anisotropic. This results in relatively thick slices in comparison with the in-plane resolution, leading to partial volume artifact.[31] Anisotropic voxels preclude the images from being reformatted into various oblique planes. As a result of the slice gaps, cartilage volume and other important structure quantifications cannot be performed accurately.

The recent introduction of an isotropic 3-dimensional (3D) imaging technique by various

Table 1
Suggested MR imaging protocol for wrist imaging at 3T (wrist coil)

Sequence	FOV (cm)	TR	TE	Slice Thickness (mm)[a]	Matrix
Cor T2 FS	8	5500	55	2.0	416 224
Ax T2 FS	8	5000	55	2.8	416 224
Cor PD FS	8	4000	35	2.0	384 192
Cor T1	8	750	20	2.0	416 192
Ax T1	8	750	20	2.8	416 192
Sag PD FS	8	4000	40	2.5	320 224
Cor CUBE Flex	12	2000	25	2	224 224

[a] No interslice gap is used on any sequences, allowing for contiguous images.

manufacturers has shown much promise in visualization of anatomy and pathology, as well as in cartilage quantification (**Table 3**). Imaging of small joints, such as the wrist and elbow, can benefit considerably from these methods. Isotropic imaging eliminates slice gaps and reduces partial volume artifact by obtaining thin contiguous slices.[32,33] The use of isotropic voxels allows images to be reformatted retrospectively into arbitrary planes to better visualize oblique anatomy (**Fig. 9**).[34] A significant decrease in scan time results as reformats can be manipulated from only 1 acquisition, as opposed to the multiplane acquisitions necessary with 2D-FSE. On the other hand, 3D-FSE scans can be limited by blurring, although extended echo trains are making this technique more feasible. Although still under development, isotropic imaging of the wrist and elbow shows promising results.

ORTHOPEDIC HARDWARE IMAGING

Metallic implants are increasingly common in the aging population. Although joint replacements are uncommon in the wrist and elbow, metallic fracture fixation hardware is frequently encountered. CT is

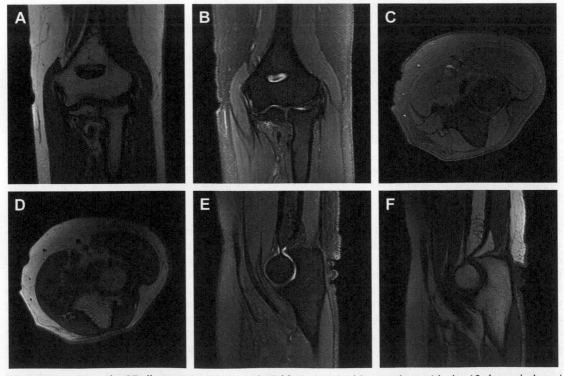

Fig. 6. Images from the 3T elbow protocol shown in **Table 3**, acquired in a patient with the 16-channel phased array flex coil. (*A*) Coronal T1-weighted image. (*B*) Coronal proton-density-weighted (PD) with fat saturation (FS) image. (*C*) Axial PD FS image. (*D*) Axial T1-weighted image. (*E*) Sagittal PD FS image. (*F*) Sagittal T1-weighted image.

Table 2
Suggested MR imaging protocol for elbow imaging at 3T

Sequence	FOV (cm)	TR	TE	Slice Thickness (mm)ᵃ	Matrix
Cor T1	14	750	17	2.0	384 192
Cor T2 FS	14	5000	55	2.0	384 224
Ax T1	14	750	17	3.0	384 192
Ax PD FS	14	4600	34	3.0	384 224
Sag T1	14	750	17	2.5	384 192
Sag T2 FS	14	4500	55	2.5	384 224

ᵃ No interslice gap is used on any sequences, allowing for contiguous images.

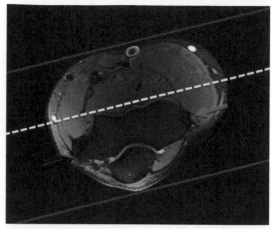

Fig. 8. Prescription for coronal images of the elbow. Select a plane along the anterior aspect of the humerus (*yellow line*) at the level of the medial (*blue arrow*) and lateral (*orange arrow*) condyles. The field of view extends to the volar and dorsal skin surfaces (*red lines*).

useful for postoperative patient monitoring and evaluating painful implants. CT, however, results in beam hardening artifacts and is insensitive to marrow edema. MR imaging has shown the most promising results in imaging orthopedic hardware because it allows for cross-sectional imaging and flexible soft tissue contrast. That said, MR imaging is also not ideal, because it suffers from imperfect corrections and susceptibility induced artifacts and signal voids. There are several factors that must be considered to optimize MR imaging for imaging around orthopedic hardware.

Simple modifications can be made to improve MR imaging around metal. For instance, gradient

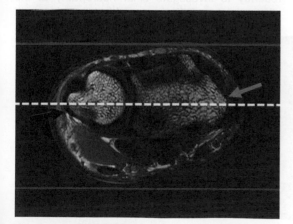

Fig. 7. Prescription for coronal images of the wrist. Select a plane (*yellow line*) parallel to the ulnar styloid (*blue arrow*) and radial styloid (*orange arrow*). The field of view extends to the volar and dorsal skin surfaces (*red lines*).

echo imaging of the soft tissue adjacent to metal is nearly impossible given the local field inhomogeneity resulting in rapid dephasing and corresponding signal voids. FSE or turbo spin-echo imaging with maximum receiver bandwidth is the preferred technique, but spatially dependent artifacts are still present.[35]

Several alternative techniques have been proposed to improve MR imaging around metal. When looking for homogenous fat suppression around the hardware, IDEAL FSE imaging has proven more reliable than fat saturation, because slowly to moderately varying field inhomogeneity can be corrected in the reconstruction.[36–38] IDEAL is a Dixon-based method for separating water and fat that allows for water-only and fat-only images to be obtained in the presence of the inhomogeneity caused by the hardware. In addition, T1-weighted images after gadolinium with water/fat separation can be acquired. Because it requires 3 acquisitions, IDEAL results in an increase in examination time; however, this can be offset with the use of parallel imaging or protocol modification.

Prepolarized MR imaging has been shown to be a promising technique to reduce artifacts around hardware.[39,40] This new, inexpensive approach to MR imaging consists of 2 electromagnets; one is a homogenous low-field readout magnet, and the second is a high-field polarizing magnet that can be somewhat inhomogeneous. This system creates 2 dynamic magnetic fields: a polarizing field, which creates the sample magnetization, and a readout field, which determines the acquisition frequency. As opposed to the traditional single

Table 3
Sequences from various manufacturers

Manufacturer	3D-Fast Spin Echo	Steady-State Free-Precession	Gradient Echo
General Electric	CUBE	GRASS	SPGR
Siemens	SPACE	FISP	FLASH
Philips	VISTA	FFE	T1 FFE

The names of 3D-Fast Spin Echo, Steady-State Free-Precession, and Gradient Echo sequences listed by manufacturer.

static magnetic field, these dual dynamic magnetic fields provide the advantage of a low field read-out that results in shift reduction of about 30-fold.[41] Prepolarized MR imaging, although helpful in resolving several of the issues that arise when imaging around metal, is not yet available clinically.

Two innovative techniques in the area of multispectral MR imaging have been developed to improve imaging around metal. Slice encoding for metal artifact correction (SEMAC) and multiple-acquisition with variable resonances image combination (MAVRIC) have exhibited great potential in correcting metal artifact. The SEMAC technique is achieved by combining view-angle tilting for correction of in-plane artifacts[42] with additional phase encoding steps in the slice dimension to fully resolve slice selective distortions.[43]

The MAVRIC technique decreases encoding errors by using several spectrally unique 3D acquisitions. MAVRIC collects several acquisitions at different frequencies to construct an image of the whole implant region. Because MAVRIC does not use slice or slab selection gradients, the spins within a MAVRIC subimage experience bandwidths determined only by the spectral properties of the applied RF pulses. The Gaussian refocusing pulses, applied with slight overlap between adjacent subimages, used in MAVRIC produce a flat sum of squares spectral response, which allow construction of the composite MAVRIC image.[44]

Although artifact reduction is quite noticeable, minor residual artifacts are still present in both the SEMAC and MAVRIC techniques. These artifacts result from using different RF pulses and spectral properties as well as a slice-selective gradient in SEMAC. Both techniques have demonstrated compatibility with partial Fourier techniques and autocalibrated parallel imaging to decrease examination time.[45,46] Although still primarily in the research stage, both SEMAC and MAVRIC allow visualization of anatomy in close proximity to metallic implants with significantly decreased artifact at reasonable examination times (**Fig. 10**).

DIFFUSION IMAGING

Diffusion-weighted imaging is increasing in popularity for body and musculoskeletal applications of MR imaging. This method has shown promise in the wrist to evaluate synovitis and bone erosions in rheumatoid arthritis.[47] It has also been used recently to investigate ulnar neuropathy at the elbow joint.[48] Diffusion-weighted imaging and

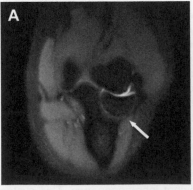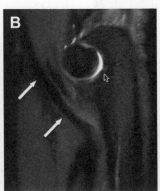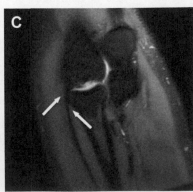

Fig. 9. Images of the elbow in a 21-year-old healthy female volunteer showing the ability of the 3D-FSE (TR/TE, 3000/35) imaging technique to visualize obliquely oriented structures in the elbow. (*A*) Oblique axial reformat illustrating the lateral ulnar collateral ligament (*arrow*). (*B*) Oblique sagittal reformat depicting the full length of the biceps tendon as well as the insertion on the same image (*arrows*). (*C*) Oblique coronal reformat illustrating the common flexor origin and the tendons that originate from it (*arrows*).

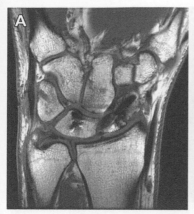
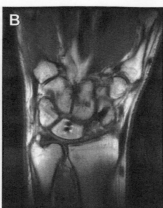

Fig. 10. Coronal T1 (*A*) and coronal PD MAVRIC (*B*) images show screw fixation of a scaphoid waist fracture. (*B*) Improved visualization of the proximal pole of the scaphoid, which is particularly important given the clinical concern for osteonecrosis.

diffusion tensor imaging are also used to evaluate articular cartilage.[49]

ULTRASHORT TE IMAGING

Ultrashort TE (uTE) imaging of the wrist and elbow shows promise in evaluation of structures that are difficult to assess on conventional MR imaging owing to short T2 relaxation times. Although tissues such as the liver and white matter have long T2 values, short T2 values ranging from hundreds of microseconds to tens of milliseconds have been recorded in ligaments, tendons, menisci, cortical bone, and periosteum.[50] uTE imaging sequences use TEs that are 20 to 50 times shorter than those used in conventional imaging sequences to detect signal changes from tissues with intrinsically short T2s.[51–53] Through this method, uTE is able to acquire a high signal from tissues that would typically produce little to no signal, such as the triangular fibrocartilage, ligamentous entheses, and trabecular bone.[54] It must be noted, however, that scan times can be considerable and slice selection can be challenging. Despite these drawbacks, uTE imaging technology provides a new approach with considerable imaging potential for the wrist and elbow.

T2 AND T1RHO MAPPING

T2 relaxation time changes obtained with spin-echo or FSE MR imaging can be quantified by using a number of T2 mapping methods. In the wrist, T2 mapping has been used to evaluate the collagen matrix status of the triangular fibrocartilage to detect early degeneration.[55] T2 relaxation time mapping is also useful to evaluate the collagen status of the articular cartilage,[56] although the elbow and wrist are studied less commonly. The median nerve signal is also

evaluated with T2 mapping[57] in the assessment of carpal tunnel syndrome. In the elbow, T2 mapping may be done to evaluate cartilage on the capitellum or trochlea.[58]

T1rho imaging, or spin-lattice relaxation in the rotating frame, has been demonstrated to be effective in visualizing proteoglycan depletion in cartilage that is associated with early osteoarthritis.[59,60] In the wrist, T1rho imaging was recently studied to evaluate degeneration of the triangular fibrocartilage.[55]

IMAGING OF WRIST MOTION

MR imaging of motion in the wrist can be done with rapid acquisition times in a single plane using real-time MR imaging.[61] Alternatively, repetitive motion cycles can be used to acquire 3D data about the motion of the carpal bones.[62] Cine phase-contrast MR imaging can also be used to determine joint motion and velocity of the carpal bones from repetitive motions in the wrist.[63] In the elbow, Cine phase-contrast MR has been used to evaluate muscle motion and contraction patterns during elbow flexion.[64]

SUMMARY

MR imaging has long been established as the preferred modality for evaluating the wrist and elbow. Technical advances in coil technology and high field scanners have improved resolution, imaging speed, and image quality. Imaging protocols should be adjusted to take advantage of advances in MR hardware and software (**Fig. 11**) to achieve high quality examinations. Newer quantitative methods such as T1rho and T2 mapping, and uTE imaging are promising techniques for evaluating earlier stages of pathology in the soft tissues.

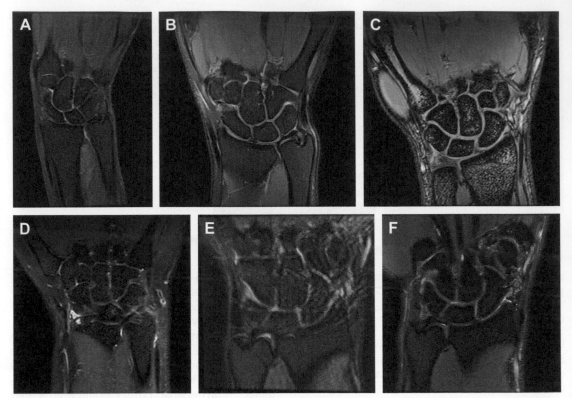

Fig. 11. Representative images of not recommended and recommended MR imaging protocols. Low-resolution not recommended. (*A*) Coronal image of the wrist using a 16 cm field of view (FOV) and a 224 × 128 matrix, 3 mm slice thickness. High-resolution recommended protocol (*B*) using a 10-cm FOV, 384 × 192 matrix, and 2 mm slice thickness. Coronal 3D gradient echo acquisition (*C*) is inferior for bone marrow lesions and ligament tears, and not recommended compared with newer 3D spin-echo based methods such as 3D FSE Cube (*D*). Uncomfortable positioning of the joint can lead to subject discomfort and motion (*E*), which can be corrected with repositioning the joint in a more comfortable location (*F*).

REFERENCES

1. Ahn JM, El-Khoury GY. Role of magnetic resonance imaging in musculoskeletal trauma. Top Magn Reson Imaging 2007;18:155–68.
2. Gold GE, Hargreaves BA, Beaulieu CF. Protocols in sports magnetic resonance imaging. Top Magn Reson Imaging 2003;14:3–23.
3. Mosher TJ. Musculoskeletal imaging at 3T: current techniques and future applications. Magn Reson Imaging Clin N Am 2006;14:63–76.
4. Kan JH. Major pitfalls in musculoskeletal imaging-MRI. Pediatr Radiol 2008;38(Suppl 2):S251–5.
5. Standaert CJ, Herring SA. Expert opinion and controversies in musculoskeletal and sports medicine: stingers. Arch Phys Med Rehabil 2009;90:402–6.
6. Pedersen JK, Lorenzen T, Ejbjerg B, et al. Low-field magnetic resonance imaging or combined ultrasonography and anti-cyclic citrullinated peptide antibody improve correct classification of individuals as established rheumatoid arthritis: results of a population-based, cross-sectional study. BMC Musculoskelet Disord 2014;15:268.
7. Suzuki T, Horikoshi M, Sugihara M, et al. Therapeutic efficacy of tocilizumab in patients with rheumatoid arthritis refractory to anti-tumor-necrosis-factor inhibitors: 1 year follow-up with low-field extremity MRI. Mod Rheumatol 2013;23:782–7.
8. Nikken JJ, Oei EH, Ginai AZ, et al. Acute peripheral joint injury: cost and effectiveness of low-field-strength MR imaging–results of randomized controlled trial. Radiology 2005;236:958–67.
9. Chang G, Friedrich KM, Wang L, et al. MRI of the wrist at 7 tesla using an eight-channel array coil combined with parallel imaging: preliminary results. J Magn Reson Imaging 2010;31:740–6.
10. Craig JG, Go L, Blechinger J, et al. Three-tesla imaging of the knee: initial experience. Skeletal Radiol 2005;34:453–61.
11. Gold GE, Han E, Stainsby J, et al. Musculoskeletal MRI at 3.0 T: relaxation times and image contrast. AJR Am J Roentgenol 2004;183:343–51.

12. Uematsu H, Takahashi M, Dougherty L, et al. High field body MR imaging: preliminary experiences. Clin Imaging 2004;28:159–62.

13. Collins CM, Smith MB. Signal-to-noise ratio and absorbed power as functions of main magnetic field strength, and definition of "90 degrees " RF pulse for the head in the birdcage coil. Magn Reson Med 2001;45:684–91.

14. Brix G, Seebass M, Hellwig G, et al. Estimation of heat transfer and temperature rise in partial-body regions during MR procedures: an analytical approach with respect to safety considerations. Magn Reson Imaging 2002;20:65–76.

15. Shellock FG. Radiofrequency energy-induced heating during MR procedures: a review. J Magn Reson Imaging 2000;12:30–6.

16. Shellock FG, Crues JV. MR procedures: biologic effects, safety, and patient care. Radiology 2004;232: 635–52.

17. Shellock FG, Spinazzi A. MRI safety update 2008: part 2, screening patients for MRI. AJR Am J Roentgenol 2008;191:1140–9.

18. Banerjee S, Krug R, Carballido-Gamio J, et al. Rapid in vivo musculoskeletal MR with parallel imaging at 7T. Magn Reson Med 2008;59:655–60.

19. Regatte RR, Schweitzer ME. Ultra-high-field MRI of the musculoskeletal system at 7.0T. J Magn Reson Imaging 2007;25:262–9.

20. Pipe JG. Motion correction with PROPELLER MRI: application to head motion and free-breathing cardiac imaging. Magn Reson Med 1999;42:963–9.

21. Reeder SB, Yu H, Johnson JW, et al. T1- and T2-weighted fast spin-echo imaging of the brachial plexus and cervical spine with IDEAL water-fat separation. J Magn Reson Imaging 2006;24: 825–32.

22. Fuller S, Reeder S, Shimakawa A, et al. Iterative decomposition of water and fat with echo asymmetry and least-squares estimation (IDEAL) fast spin-echo imaging of the ankle: initial clinical experience. AJR Am J Roentgenol 2006;187:1442–7.

23. Cerezal L, Llopis E, Canga A, et al. MR arthrography of the ankle: indications and technique. Radiol Clin North Am 2008;46:973–94, v.

24. Morrison WB. Indirect MR arthrography: concepts and controversies. Semin Musculoskelet Radiol 2005;9:125–34.

25. Bergin D, Schweitzer ME. Indirect magnetic resonance arthrography. Skeletal Radiol 2003;32:551–8.

26. Zlatkin MB, Pevsner D, Sanders TG, et al. Acetabular labral tears and cartilage lesions of the hip: indirect MR arthrographic correlation with arthroscopy–a preliminary study. AJR Am J Roentgenol 2010;194:709–14.

27. Steinbach LS, Palmer WE, Schweitzer ME. Special focus session. MR arthrography. Radiographics 2002;22:1223–46.

28. Jee WH, McCauley TR, Kim JM, et al. Meniscal tear configurations: categorization with MR imaging. AJR Am J Roentgenol 2003;180:93–7.

29. Schaefer FK, Schaefer PJ, Brossmann J, et al. Value of fat-suppressed PD-weighted TSE-sequences for detection of anterior and posterior cruciate ligament lesions–comparison to arthroscopy. Eur J Radiol 2006;58:411–5.

30. Sonin AH, Pensy RA, Mulligan ME, et al. Grading articular cartilage of the knee using fast spin-echo proton density-weighted MR imaging without fat suppression. AJR Am J Roentgenol 2002;179: 1159–66.

31. Bredella MA, Tirman PF, Peterfy CG, et al. Accuracy of T2-weighted fast spin-echo MR imaging with fat saturation in detecting cartilage defects in the knee: comparison with arthroscopy in 130 patients. AJR Am J Roentgenol 1999;172:1073–80.

32. Gold GE, Busse RF, Beehler C, et al. Isotropic MRI of the knee with 3D fast spin-echo extended echo-train acquisition (XETA): initial experience. AJR Am J Roentgenol 2007;188:1287–93.

33. Lichy MP, Wietek BM, Mugler JP 3rd, et al. Magnetic resonance imaging of the body trunk using a single-slab, 3-dimensional, T2-weighted turbo-spin-echo sequence with high sampling efficiency (SPACE) for high spatial resolution imaging: initial clinical experiences. Invest Radiol 2005;40:754–60.

34. Stevens KJ, Busse RF, Han E, et al. Ankle: isotropic MR imaging with 3D-FSE-cube–initial experience in healthy volunteers. Radiology 2008;249:1026–33.

35. Butts K, Pauly JM, Gold GE. Reduction of blurring in view angle tilting MRI. Magn Reson Med 2005;53: 418–24.

36. Kijowski R, Blankenbaker DG, Woods MA, et al. 3.0-T evaluation of knee cartilage by using three-dimensional IDEAL GRASS imaging: comparison with fast spin-echo imaging. Radiology 2010;255: 117–27.

37. Chen CA, Lu W, John CT, et al. Multiecho IDEAL gradient-echo water-fat separation for rapid assessment of cartilage volume at 1.5 T: initial experience. Radiology 2009;252:561–7.

38. Gold GE, Reeder SB, Yu H, et al. Articular cartilage of the knee: rapid three-dimensional MR imaging at 3.0 T with IDEAL balanced steady-state free precession–initial experience. Radiology 2006;240:546–51.

39. Kegler C, Seton HC, Hutchison JM. Prepolarized fast spin-echo pulse sequence for low-field MRI. Magn Reson Med 2007;57:1180–4.

40. Venook RD, Matter NI, Ramachandran M, et al. Prepolarized magnetic resonance imaging around metal orthopedic implants. Magn Reson Med 2006;56:177–86.

41. Morgan P, Conolly S, Scott G, et al. A readout magnet for prepolarized MRI. Magn Reson Med 1996;36: 527–36.

42. Cho ZH, Kim DJ, Kim YK. Total inhomogeneity correction including chemical shifts and susceptibility by view angle tilting. Med Phys 1988;15:7–11.

43. Lu W, Pauly KB, Gold GE, et al. SEMAC: slice encoding for metal artifact correction in MRI. Magn Reson Med 2009;62:66–76.

44. Koch KM, Lorbiecki JE, Hinks RS, et al. A multispectral three-dimensional acquisition technique for imaging near metal implants. Magn Reson Med 2009;61:381–90.

45. Chen W, Beatty P, Koch KM, et al. Parallel MRI near metallic implants. 17th Annual Meeting of the ISMRM. Honolulu, HI, April 18–24, 2009. p. 2783.

46. Lu W, Pauly KB, Gold GE, et al. Accelerated slice-encoding for metal artifact correction. 17th Annual ISMRM. Honolulu, HI, April 18–24, 2009. p. 258.

47. Li X, Liu X, Du X, et al. Diffusion-weighted MR imaging for assessing synovitis of wrist and hand in patients with rheumatoid arthritis: a feasibility study. Magn Reson Imaging 2014;32:350–3.

48. Altun Y, Aygun MS, Cevik MU, et al. Relation between electrophysiological findings and diffusion weighted magnetic resonance imaging in ulnar neuropathy at the elbow. J Neuroradiol 2013;40:260–6.

49. Staroswiecki E, Granlund K, Alley M, et al. Diffusion-weighted imaging and T2-maps of knee cartilage with a DESS sequence at 3T. Stockholm (Sweden): International Society for Magnetic Resonance in Medicine OISMRM); 2010.

50. Gatehouse PD, Thomas RW, Robson MD, et al. Magnetic resonance imaging of the knee with ultrashort TE pulse sequences. Magn Reson Imaging 2004;22:1061–7.

51. Gatehouse PD, He T, Puri BK, et al. Contrast-enhanced MRI of the menisci of the knee using ultrashort echo time (UTE) pulse sequences: imaging of the red and white zones. Br J Radiol 2004;77:641–7.

52. Gold GE, Thedens DR, Pauly JM, et al. MR imaging of articular cartilage of the knee: new methods using ultrashort TEs. AJR Am J Roentgenol 1998;170:1223–6.

53. Robson MD, Gatehouse PD, Bydder M, et al. Magnetic resonance: an introduction to ultrashort TE (UTE) imaging. J Comput Assist Tomogr 2003;27:825–46.

54. Wurnig MC, Calcagni M, Kenkel D, et al. Characterization of trabecular bone density with ultra-short echo-time MRI at 1.5, 3.0 and 7.0 T–comparison with micro-computed tomography. NMR Biomed 2014;27:1159–66.

55. Rauscher I, Bender B, Grozinger G, et al. Assessment of T1, T1rho, and T2 values of the ulnocarpal disc in healthy subjects at 3 tesla. Magn Reson Imaging 2014;32:1085–90.

56. Mosher TJ, Smith H, Dardzinski BJ, et al. MR imaging and T2 mapping of femoral cartilage: in vivo determination of the magic angle effect. AJR Am J Roentgenol 2001;177:665–9.

57. Cha JG, Han JK, Im SB, et al. Median nerve T2 assessment in the wrist joints: preliminary study in patients with carpal tunnel syndrome and healthy volunteers. J Magn Reson Imaging 2014;40:789–95.

58. Wucherer KL, Ober CP, Conzemius MG. The use of delayed gadolinium enhanced magnetic resonance imaging of cartilage and T2 mapping to evaluate articular cartilage in the normal canine elbow. Vet Radiol Ultrasound 2012;53:57–63.

59. Akella SV, Regatte RR, Gougoutas AJ, et al. Proteoglycan-induced changes in T1rho-relaxation of articular cartilage at 4T. Magn Reson Med 2001;46:419–23.

60. Li X, Han ET, Ma CB, et al. In vivo 3T spiral imaging based multi-slice T(1rho) mapping of knee cartilage in osteoarthritis. Magn Reson Med 2005;54:929–36.

61. Boutin RD, Buonocore MH, Immerman I, et al. Real-time magnetic resonance imaging (MRI) during active wrist motion–initial observations. PLoS One 2013;8:e84004.

62. Moritomo H, Murase T, Goto A, et al. In vivo three-dimensional kinematics of the midcarpal joint of the wrist. J Bone Joint Surg Am 2006;88:611–21.

63. Behnam AJ, Herzka DA, Sheehan FT. Assessing the accuracy and precision of musculoskeletal motion tracking using cine-PC MRI on a 3.0T platform. J Biomech 2011;44:193–7.

64. Pappas GP, Asakawa DS, Delp SL, et al. Nonuniform shortening in the biceps brachii during elbow flexion. J Appl Physiol (1985) 2002;92:2381–9.

MR Imaging of Wrist Ligaments

Michael D. Ringler, MD*, Naveen S. Murthy, MD

KEYWORDS

- MR imaging wrist • MRI wrist • Wrist ligaments • Scapholunate • Lunotriquetral
- Extrinsic ligaments • Intrinsic ligaments • Diagnostic performance • Carpal instability

KEY POINTS

- Ligamentous injury to the wrist is a common cause of chronic wrist pain and carpal instability.
- MR imaging, coupled with knowledge of normal anatomy, allows consistent visualization of all major intrinsic and extrinsic wrist ligaments.
- Ligament tears are diagnosed by the presence of abnormal signal hyperintensity on fluid-sensitive sequences, ligament discontinuity, or altered morphology.
- MR imaging has excellent specificity, good sensitivity, and substantial interobserver agreement for diagnosis of partial and complete scapholunate and lunotriquetral ligament tears. Sensitivity is enhanced with higher field strengths and use of magnetic resonance arthrography.
- Appropriate clinical management is guided by wrist MR imaging interpretation.

DISCUSSION OF THE PROBLEM

There is a high prevalence of ligamentous injury to the wrist in the setting of trauma, particularly in the presence of bone abnormalities.[1–4] A recent study found that 60% of patients presenting for wrist MR imaging following trauma had intrinsic ligament injury and 75% had extrinsic ligament injury.[4] Such traumatic ligament injuries have delayed functional consequences[5] such as progressive carpal instability with secondary deterioration of the wrist joint and chronic wrist pain.[6–8] However, a history of trauma is not always elicited, and this has led to the theory that, in some cases, degenerative changes in ligaments alone may cause pain in the stable wrist,[9–11] and may extend over time, possibly via increased local motion, to complete tears and resultant instability.[12] Regardless of cause, appropriate clinical management is predicated on accurate and timely diagnosis.[13,14]

MR imaging is a proven, established technology for the detection, evaluation, and follow-up of disorders of the wrist, including ligamentous disorders.[14–16] Wrist MR imaging frequently alters planned clinical management, including the decision to perform surgery.[14] All of the major intrinsic and extrinsic wrist ligaments are easily identified[17–25] on 1.5 T and 3 T MR imaging with a range of accuracies for tear detection depending on the particular ligament and disorder type.[7,26–36] MR imaging is considered appropriate in the work-up of both radial-sided and ulnar-sided wrist pain with normal or nonspecific radiographs, according to the American College of Radiology Appropriateness Criteria.[37]

ANATOMY

The ligaments of the wrist guide and constrain the complex motion of the carpus relative to the forearm and metacarpals, and facilitate transmission of force between carpal bones.[38–40] They are commonly divided into intrinsic and extrinsic groups.[41] Intrinsic ligaments arise and insert

Disclosure: The Authors have nothing to disclose.
Department of Radiology, Mayo Clinic, 200 First Street Southwest, Rochester, MN 55905, USA
* Corresponding author.
E-mail address: ringler.michael@mayo.edu

1064-9689/15/$ – see front matter © 2015 Elsevier Inc. All rights reserved.

mri.theclinics.com

entirely within the carpus onto carpal bones, whereas extrinsic ligaments arise in the forearm, or extend onto metacarpals, and have additional attachments to retinacula and/or tendon sheaths.[41,42] The appropriate nomenclature is to name the ligaments for the bones from which they originate and onto which they insert, proximal to distal, radial to ulnar.[43] This article describes some of the most important ligaments organized by anatomic location.

Interosseous Ligaments

Interosseous ligaments are intrinsic intercarpal ligaments that unite carpal bones either within a carpal row or between carpal rows. The most important and well-studied are those that separate the radiocarpal and midcarpal compartments, providing the flexible linkage of the proximal carpal row, the scapholunate ligament (SLL) and lunotriquetral ligament (LTT).[42,44] In contradistinction, the 3 distal carpal row interosseous ligaments that unite the trapezium with the trapezoid, the trapezoid with the capitate, and the capitate with the hamate, allow normal communication between the midcarpal and common carpometacarpal compartments, as they do not extend from volar wrist joint capsule to dorsal capsule.[44]

Scapholunate ligament

The SLL is a C-shaped[39] structure, approximately 18 mm in length, and 2 to 3 mm in thickness,[12] connecting the mutually articulating surfaces of the ulnar scaphoid and radial lunate (**Fig. 1**).[45] It has 3 histologically and functionally distinct segments.[45] Knowledge of segmental anatomy is crucial because the site and extent of the ligament disruption may be used to differentiate between a traumatic tear and a degenerative perforation, the latter of which sometimes represents asymptomatic senescent change.[31,46]

Dorsal scapholunate ligament

The dorsal segment of the SLL is a true histologic articular ligament, with normally taut transversely oriented collagen fascicles averaging 3 to 5 mm in proximal to distal length (**Fig. 1**).[45] It has a trapezoidal shape in the axial plane, with shorter volar fibers, and is intimately associated with the dorsal joint capsule. Distally it merges with the dorsal intercarpal ligament (DIL).[45]

Volar scapholunate ligament

The volar segment of the SLL is a much thinner ligament (no more than 1 mm thick), with slightly obliquely oriented collagen fibers from proximal-ulnar to distal-radial.[45] The lunate attachment is just dorsal to

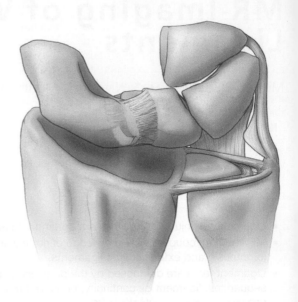

Fig. 1. Interosseous ligament. Note the 3 histologically and functionally distinct segments of the SLL, with meniscoid proximal fibrocartilaginous component, and transversely oriented collagenous dorsal and volar components. The LTL is analogous (not shown). Capsular ligaments have been removed. (*From* Mayo Foundation for Medical Education and Research, all rights reserved; with permission.)

the long radiolunate ligament (LRL) attachment and immediately proximal to the cartilage surface. It is not normally possible to directly visualize the volar SLL with an arthroscope, because thin laminae of collagen fibers extending from the radioscapholunate neurovascular bundle isolate it from the radiocarpal joint.[45]

Proximal (membranous) scapholunate ligament

Unlike the dorsal and volar segments of the SLL, the proximal or membranous segment is grossly anisotropic fibrocartilage rather than a true ligament.[45] It has a pliable consistency and its attachments blend with the articular cartilage of the scaphoid and lunate. Usually there is a meniscus-like extension that protrudes into the scapholunate joint space, with wedge-shaped or triangular cross-sectional geometry, usually nicely shown in the coronal pane with MR imaging (**Fig. 1**).[12,45] This segment is the weakest part of the SLL, prone to degenerative perforations, and the only area of the SLL that can be readily seen by arthroscopy in the absence of scapholunate dissocation.[12]

Lunotriquetral ligament

The lunotriquetral ligament (LTL) is slightly longer, measuring approximately 20 mm in length, and more V shaped than the SLL; however, it also has 3 histologically and functionally distinct segments.[12,47] The LTL segments could be viewed as the reverse of the SLL segments, in that the volar LTL is thicker and potentially more important than the dorsal LTL, whereas the dorsal SLL is thicker than the volar SLL.[38]

Dorsal lunotriquetral ligament The dorsal segment of the LTL is a true histologic ligament with transverse collagenous fibers, measuring up to only 1 to 1.5 mm in thickness, making it challenging to identify on MR imaging.[12] It is covered by the dorsal radiocarpal ligament (DRL).[38]

Volar lunotriquetral ligament The volar region is the thickest segment, composed of transversely oriented collagen fascicles that interweave with the ulnocapitate ligament (UCL), measuring up to 2.5 mm in thickness.[48] It transmits the extension moment of the triquetrum.[40]

Proximal (membranous lunotriquetral ligament) Similar to the proximal SLL, the proximal LTL is composed of fibrocartilage and often shows a meniscal projection into the lunotriquetral joint.[38] However, it is much thinner than the proximal SLL, often no more than 1 to 1.5 mm, which has made it unreliable to visualize on MR imaging in the past.[12]

Scaphotrapeziotrapezoid ligament
The scaphotrapeziotrapezoid ligament (STL) is composed of collagenous fibers that span the volar and dorsal aspects of the distal pole of the scaphoid and proximal trapezium with some fibers extending to the trapezoid.[42] Some fibers from the radioscaphocapitate ligament (RSL) blend with the volar STL, which is not visible arthroscopically.[42,50]

Volar Capsular Ligaments

Volar radiocarpal ligaments
These extrinsic extrasynovial capsular ligaments span the width of the palmar rim of the distal radius and attach distally to carpal bones (**Fig. 2**).[8,38] They play roles in preventing ulnar translation of the carpus,[51] and secondary stabilization of the scaphoid and lunate.[44,52] The osseous attachments cannot be directly visualized with multiportal wrist arthroscopy.[2,6]

Radial collateral ligament The radial collateral ligament (RCL), or radioscaphoid ligament, runs from the radial styloid process to the scaphoid tuberosity and the flexor carpi radialis tendon (**Fig. 2**).[44] It is sometimes considered part of the RSL rather than a separate structure.[53]

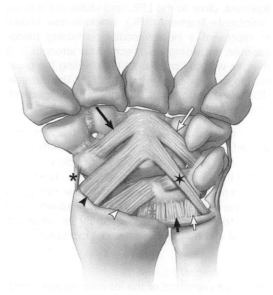

Fig. 2. Volar capsular ligaments. RCL (*black asterisk*), RSL (*black arrowhead*), LRL (*white arrowhead*), SRL (*red asterisk*), ULL (*short black arrow*), UTL (*short white arrow*), UCL (*star*), radial limb (SCL) of arcuate ligament (*long black arrow*), and ulnar limb (THL) of arcuate ligament (*long white arrow*). (From Mayo Foundation for Medical Education and Research, all rights reserved; with permission.)

Radioscaphocapitate ligament The RSL arises from the tip of the radial styloid process through the middle of the scaphoid fossa, supports the waist of the scaphoid, attaches to the proximal cortex of the distal scaphoid pole, and distally interdigitates with fibers from the UCL and palmar scaphotriquetral ligament, with only about 10% of fibers ultimately inserting on the capitate (**Fig. 2**).[38] This ligament plays a role in scaphoid stability,[52] acting as a sling or "seat belt" at the scaphoid waist.[8] In general, it is easily seen on arthroscopy, except for the radial styloid attachment and where it crosses the scaphoid waist, making tears in these areas difficult to diagnose.[34,54]

Long radiolunate ligament The LRL, also known as the radiolunotriquetral ligament, arises from the palmar rim of the remaining scaphoid fossa, passes anterior to the proximal scaphoid pole, and attaches to the radial volar lunate cortex (**Fig. 2**).[53] In some cases it extends in 1 continuous sheet to the triquetrum[55] or it may exist as 2 separate radiolunate and lunotriquetral portions, with superficial fibers blending with the LTL.[53] It serves as a volar sling for the lunate.[44]

Radioscapholunate bundle At one time there was a structure described as the radioscapholunate ligament, ulnar to the LRL, and radial to the short radiolunate ligament (SRL), which is now known to represent a neurovascular-containing meso-capsule, providing no mechanical strength.[56] It merges with the proximal SLL, dividing the prox-imal from volar segments (**Fig. 3**).[45] The term ra-dioscapholunate bundle, rather than ligament, may be preferred.[25]

Short radiolunate ligament The SRL arises from the entire width of the volar rim of the lunate fossa of the radius and attaches distally onto the radial half of the lunate volar cortex (**Fig. 2**).[53] The lunate is therefore strongly anchored to the radius via both the LRL and SRL, which may explain why it tends to remain in place despite the traumatic force of a complete perilunate dislocation.[38]

Volar midcarpal ligaments

The most important of the intrinsic capsular mid-carpal ligaments include the arcuate and deltoid ligament complexes. Both form a V, flanking the proximal normal zone of volar capsular deficiency, in the carpal tunnel floor, known as the space of Poirier, through which volar lunate dislocation oc-curs.[18,43,44,57] Although technically separate struc-tures, particularly proximally, the arcuate and deltoid ligaments blend imperceptibly with each other as they approach their common attachment on the capitate, making them practically indistin-guishable distally.[20] In the literature, the arcuate

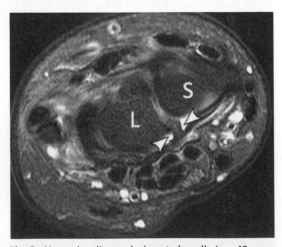

Fig. 3. Normal radioscapholunate bundle in a 40-year-old woman with chronic, intermittent ulnar wrist pain. Axial T2-weighted fat-saturated image shows the normal radioscapholunate bundle (*arrowheads*) attaching to the junction of the volar and proximal segments of the SLL. Scaphoid (S) and lunate (L) bones. Note the low-signal ligamentous appearance of this neurovascular-containing mesocapsule.

ligament is sometimes referred to as the deltoid ligament[44] and the deltoid ligament referred to as the arcuate ligament.[38]

Arcuate ligament The arcuate ligament is composed of the scaphocapitate ligament (SCL) or radial limb and triquetrohamocapitate ligament (THL) or ulnar limb, neither of which are visible by arthroscopy (**Fig. 2**).[20,50] It has also been described in the radiology literature as the distal band of the palmar scaphotriquetral ligament.[4,25] The palmar scaphotriquetral ligament is another intrinsic capsular ligament extending from scaphoid to triquetrum, at the level of the midcar-pal joint, superficial to the SCL and THL.[38]

Deltoid ligament The distal RSL and UCL consti-tute radial and ulnar limbs, respectively, of the del-toid ligament.[57] Distally they form transversely oriented interdigitating fibers that support the head of the capitate in the midcarpal joint, like a labrum.[38] Fibers from the deltoid ligament also interdigitate with the palmar scaphotriquetral ligament.[38]

Volar ulnocarpal ligaments

Ulnolunate and ulnotriquetral ligaments The ul-nolunate ligament (ULL) and ulnotriquetral liga-ment (UTL) both arise proximally from the volar radioulnar ligament of the triangular fibrocartilage complex (TFCC), and form the anterior and ulnar aspects of the ulnocarpal joint capsule.[40,58] They exist as a continuous sheet, also including the SRL, without any demarcation between them, distinguished only by their distal attachments (**Fig. 2**).[38] The ULL attaches distally to the volar ul-nar cortex of the lunate, and the UTL attaches to the proximal and ulnar surfaces of the triquetrum, sometimes with a few fibers attaching to the ulnar styloid process as well.[38]

The UTL often has 2 normal perforations: a proximal opening to the prestyloid recess, and a distal pisotriquetral joint orifice.[38] The distal tri-quetral attachment of the UTL, where tears are sometimes seen on MR imaging, is difficult to see with arthroscopy.[59] The TFCC is discussed in MRI of the Triangular Fibrocartilage Complex by ME Cody, DT Nakamura, KM Small and H Yoshioka.

Ulnocapitate ligament The UCL is superficial to the other 2 ulnocarpal ligaments, and is the only one to attach directly to the ulnar head fovea.[38] It reinforces the volar LTL and then passes radi-ally and distally into the midcarpal joint to contribute to the deltoid ligament, with only about 10% of fibers directly attaching to the capitate (**Fig. 2**).[38]

Dorsal Capsular Ligaments

Early ligament sectioning studies focused on evaluation of intrinsic and volar extrinsic ligaments via dorsal approaches to elevate soft tissue flaps; however, this disrupted the dorsal capsular ligaments in the process.[60] There is now mounting evidence that the dorsal capsular ligaments of the wrist play as important a role in carpal stability as volar capsular and interosseous ligaments.[48,57,60–64] The DRL and DIL form a V with the apex pointed at their common attachment on the triquetrum (**Fig. 3**). This angle of intersection at the triquetrum goes from acute in wrist extension to nearly orthogonal in palmar flexion. It is thought that this linkage system may provide stability between the radius and scaphoid indirectly without compromising motion.[65] The osseous attachments cannot be directly visualized with multiportal wrist arthroscopy.[6]

Dorsal radiocarpal ligament

Also known as the dorsal radiotriquetral ligament, in most cases the DRL originates from the dorsal rim of the distal radius, spanning the Lister tubercle to the sigmoid notch.[38] It then passes obliquely distally and ulnarly to attach to the dorsal ulnar horn of the lunate, dorsal LTL, and fourth and fifth extensor compartment septa, and terminates just proximal to the radial dorsal ridge of the triquetrum (**Fig. 4**).[65,66] Three less common variants have

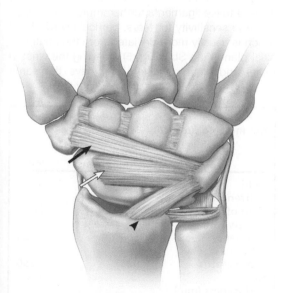

Fig. 4. Dorsal capsular ligaments. DRL (*arrowhead*), proximal fascicle of DIL (*white arrow*), and distal fascicle of DIL (*black arrow*). (*From* Mayo Foundation for Medical Education and Research, all rights reserved; with permission.)

been described, which involve either separate bands or additional radial fibers that may cover the dorsal proximal scaphoid.[65,67]

Dorsal intercarpal ligament

This intrinsic capsular ligament, also known as the dorsal scaphotriquetral ligament, inserts distal to the dorsal ridge of triquetrum on its radial aspect.[66] It then passes radially, where it attaches to the dorsal distal lunate and dorsal groove of scaphoid, with additional fibers attaching distally to the dorsal proximal rim of the trapezium in most wrists (**Fig. 4**).[23,65] In one cadaveric study, there were additional fibers from the DIL that attached to the trapezoid in 42% and the capitate in 7%.[65] The 2 most commonly described variants include a single band that branches radially to attach to the scaphoid and trapezium, and 2 distinct fascicles.[23,38]

MR IMAGING
Protocol

The salient considerations of optimal wrist MR imaging are well summarized in a practice parameter developed collaboratively by the American College of Radiology, the Society of Computed Body Tomography and Magnetic Resonance, the Society for Pediatric Radiology, and the Society of Skeletal Radiology.[16]

Depending on the clinician's needs and choice of coil, the patient can be positioned in the bore of the scanner either supine or prone. The supine position with the wrist imaged alongside the patient may be more comfortable and decrease the risk of claustrophobia.[68,69] However, because of decreased magnetic field homogeneity peripherally, image quality may suffer from decreased signal/noise ratio (SNR) or incomplete chemically selective fat saturation.[16,68] Scanning the patient prone with the upper extremity overhead, the so-called superman position, allows the wrist to be imaged in the homogenous center of the magnetic field, at the increased risk of motion artifact from potential discomfort.[68]

Thin high-resolution images are required to evaluate the small ligaments of the wrist, which often take a double-oblique course in three-dimensional (3D) space.[19] In order to achieve the requisite spatial resolution, a high SNR is required, and is achieved primarily through the use of an appropriate local receiver coil.[16,70,71] There are many different acceptable surface coil design options.[7,72–74] Without the proper coil, MR imaging cannot reliably diagnose wrist ligamentous disorders.[75] The smallest surface coils, known as microscopy coils, are less than 5 cm in diameter, show even higher SNR and contrast/noise ratio than the standard small surface coil, but have a limited field of view (FOV), precluding imaging of the entire wrist at once.[76]

A static magnetic field strength of at least 1 T is recommended.[16,74] Higher field strengths provide greater SNR, which facilitates improved visualization of wrist ligaments.[77,78] Although all of the major wrist ligaments are routinely identified at 1.5 T,[17,31,42] imaging at 3 T has additional benefits, including increased ligament conspicuity.[77,78] The additional SNR obtained from greater than 1.5 T imaging can be exploited to increase spatial resolution, obtain a larger FOV without losing spatial resolution, or scan in a shorter time period while maintaining adequate spatial resolution.[30,79]

Wrist ligaments are optimally visualized with an FOV of 6 to 8 cm, assuming there is adequate SNR available,[7,21,22,80] otherwise up to 12 cm may still allow consistent visualization of wrist ligaments and TFCC.[23,24,28,72,73,81,82] A rectangular FOV can save imaging time without sacrificing spatial resolution.[16] Higher imaging matrices are necessary for adequate spatial resolution, but are limited by available intravoxel SNR and imaging time.[83] At least 256 steps in the frequency direction and 192 steps in the phase direction for two-dimensional (2D) imaging is recommended,[16,22,80] and slice thickness should be no greater than 3 mm to minimize partial volume effects.[7,26,73,83,84] Two-dimensional fast spin echo (FSE) slices 2 mm thick are routinely obtained with 3 T magnets.[30]

The thinnest slice thicknesses obtainable, typically 0.6 to 1.2 mm, are acquired through volumetric 3D pulse sequences.[19,21,22,24,28,72,80,81] Initially these volumetric acquisitions were of the gradient echo (GRE) variety, resulting in T2*-weighted images, and thought to be most useful for assessing the interosseous ligaments because of the thin sections obtainable.[26,84] However, more recently, isotropic 3D FSE sequences have become available, which have superior SNR, in addition to the usual isotropic 3D acquisition benefits of ability to reconstruct data into any arbitrary plane with thin slice thickness.[85] However, at this time, blurring in reconstructed planes remains a problem because of T2 decay during the required long echo trains.[85] Whether obtained via 3D reconstructions or primary 2D acquisitions, oblique planes may add significant value to assessment of intrinsic and extrinsic ligaments, which also run in oblique planes.[23,24,66,86]

Fluid-sensitive pulse sequences, such as T2-weighted, T2*-weighted (GRE), short-tau inversion recovery (STIR), intermediate-weighted (long recovery time; echo time, 30–60 milliseconds), and proton density–weighted sequences, are most helpful for evaluating the wrist ligaments.[7,21,22,73,80,83] Fat suppression, whether accomplished via spectrally selective radiofrequency pulses; a phase-dependent method (Dixon technique); or, if necessary, STIR, enhances diagnostic yield (**Box 1**).[16,87–90] Gadolinium-enhanced magnetic resonance arthrography (MRA) may improve diagnostic performance for ligamentous disorders[28,72,73,83]; this is discussed in a separate article MR arthrography of the wrist and elbow by Bancroft and colleagues. In addition, a type of fast GRE pulse sequence known as balanced steady-state free precession is able to generate images rapidly enough (<0.6 seconds per image) to allow the moving wrist to be imaged.[91] This kinematic or active MR imaging pulse sequence could potentially be used to investigate dynamic carpal instability by supplementing an otherwise high-spatial-resolution examination with high-temporal-resolution images, although this has yet to be proved.[92]

Normal MR Imaging Appearance

Interosseous ligaments

Ligaments are optimally evaluated with slices oriented with respect to their long axis, or orthogonal to potential tears.[20,66,86] Therefore, although the proximal segments of SLL and LTL are best seen in the coronal plane, the dorsal and volar segments are better appreciated on the axial images.[76] Oblique axial images through the long axes of these ligaments further improve visualization and sensitivity for tears, particularly of LTL,[86] which is usually more deviated from the anatomic axial plane than SLL (**Fig. 5**). Imaging the wrist in radial and ulnar deviation may have the same

Box 1 MR imaging protocol		
	Minimal Requirements	Ideal
Field Strength (T)	1	3
Field of View (cm)	12	6–8
Frequency Matrix	256	384
Phase Matrix	192	256
Slice Thickness (mm)	3	1–2
Pulse Sequences	Fat-saturated fluid-sensitive sequences (30-60 milliscecond echo time)	

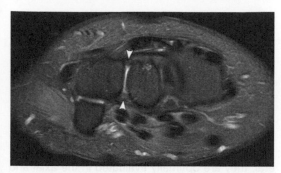

Fig. 5. Normal dorsal and volar lunotriquetral ligament segments in a 26-year-old woman with chronic dorsal wrist pain caused by injury 6 years earlier. Oblique axial T2-weighted fat-saturated image through the long axis of the lunotriquetral ligament shows normal low signal, and bandlike dorsal and volar components (*arrowheads*).

effect, with the added benefit of changes in radiocarpal joint width[93]; however, normal interosseous ligament morphology and signal may be altered with wrist position.[94]

Dorsal and volar segments

Scapholunate ligament and lunotriquetral ligament The appearance of the interosseous ligaments of the proximal carpal row vary depending on the slice thickness, spatial resolution, pulse sequence, coil, and wrist position.[76,82,94,95] Usually the dorsal and volar components of both SLL and LTL are bandlike on axial images, with predominantly low signal intensity on all pulse sequences, because of the homogeneous transversely oriented collagen fascicles (**Fig. 5**; **Fig. 6**).[17,22] However, the volar SLL often shows

striated heterogenous increased signal intensity, particularly on GRE sequences, probably related to associated loose vascular connective tissue.[22] Occasionally, the volar or dorsal SLL appears triangular on axial images, similar to the proximal SLL on coronal images, suggesting continuation of the intra-articular meniscoid component (**Fig. 6**).[12,17]

Proximal segments

Scapholunate ligament Most of the fibrocartilaginous proximal SLL has a triangular shape on coronal images and shows heterogenous, predominantly low, signal intensity.[22] It normally attaches to intermediate-signal-intensity hyaline cartilage on both the lunate and the scaphoid. Coronal slices approaching the volar SLL instead usually show a trapezoid-shaped heterogenous intermediate-signal-intensity ligament, attaching directly to cortex.[22,82,94] Coronal images approaching the dorsal SLL often show a bandlike low-signal-intensity structure variably attaching to cortex and articular cartilage (**Fig. 7**).[22,94]

Lunotriquetral ligament The proximal fibrocartilaginous LTL is also triangular on most coronal images, although it may appear more linear as the volar LTL is approached (**Fig. 7**).[76] Although initially described as having mostly homogeneous low signal intensity,[95] subsequent evaluation with higher-resolution techniques using a microscopy

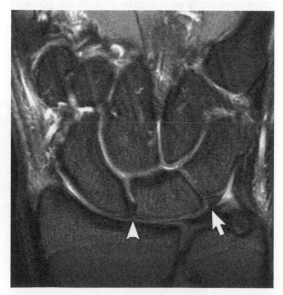

Fig. 7. Normal proximal (membranous) scapholunate and lunotriquetral ligament segments in a 17-year-old boy with wrist pain following a motor vehicle accident. Coronal T2-weighted fat-saturated image shows low-signal fibrocartilaginous meniscoid proximal components of the scapholunate (*arrowhead*) and lunotriquetral (*arrow*) ligaments.

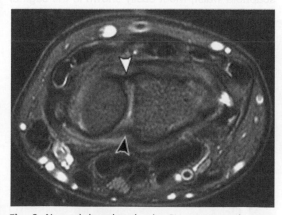

Fig. 6. Normal dorsal and volar SLL segments in a 15-year-old girl experiencing wrist pain after a difficult volleyball set the day before. Axial T2-weighted fat-saturated image shows normal low-signal dorsal (*white arrowhead*) and volar (*black arrowhead*) components of the SLL. The volar segment often has normal mildly heterogenous intermediate signal intensity.

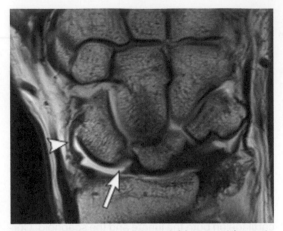

Fig. 8. Normal RCL in a 37-year-old man with persistent ulnar wrist pain after hitting punching bag a year earlier. Coronal T1-weighted image, with intraarticular gadolinium contrast agent, shows linear low-signal RCL (*arrowhead*). Also note the proximal SLL detachment from the scaphoid (*arrow*).

coil have described 3 different major types of presumed normal signal intensity.[76] The most common (45.5%) consisted of linear intermediate or high signal intensity traversing the distal surface of the proximal LTL (type 2), followed by homogeneous low signal intensity (type 1, 33.8%), followed by linear intermediate or high signal intensity traversing both proximal and distal surfaces (type 3, 20.8%).[76] An amorphous shape is more commonly seen in older individuals, possibly representing degenerative change.[76,94,95]

Scaphotrapeziotrapezoid ligament

When seen, the STL usually shows mildly heterogenous low signal intensity, with striations, on fluid-sensitive sequences. The dorsal component is reportedly more easily seen;[50] however, there is a paucity of imaging literature regarding this ligament at this time.

Volar capsular ligaments

Capsular ligaments generally appear on MR imaging as linear hypointense structures,[25] often with alternating bands of intermediate signal intensity leading to a striated appearance.[17,19,21,24] In general, they are optimally evaluated in the axial and sagittal planes, with the exception of the RCL, which is better evaluated in the axial and coronal planes.[17,25]

Radial collateral ligament The RCL is a thin, low-signal-intensity structure that arises from the tip of the radial styloid process, radial to the common origin of RSL and LRL, and inserts on the radial aspect of the scaphoid waist (**Fig. 8**).[17,25,44] It is more easily identified in the presence of a radiocarpal joint effusion, or with MRA,[17] and measures approximately 5.1 mm by 1.2 mm on average in the axial plane.[25]

Radioscaphocapitate and long radiolunate ligaments The radial and palmar origins of the RSL and LRL on the radial styloid process are intimately associated, and often cannot be distinguished on MR imaging.[17,25] Proximally they run nearly parallel and immediately adjacent to each other, the LRL proximal and ulnar to the RSL, with a fluid-signal-intensity interligamentous sulcus, sometimes visible on MR imaging (**Fig. 9**).[18,34,39] Both ligaments take a distal and ulnar oblique course, traversing a groove in the scaphoid waist, most easily shown in the sagittal

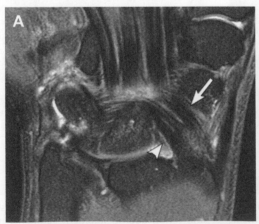
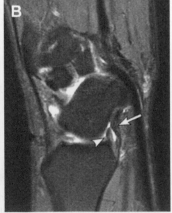

Fig. 9. Normal RSL (*arrow*) and LRL (*arrowhead*) on (*A*) coronal and (*B*) sagittal T2-weighted fat-saturated images. Like most capsular ligaments, they are predominantly low signal with linear higher-signal striations. Note the normal fluid-filled interligamentous sulcus between the 2 ligaments in (*B*). The patient in (*A*) is a 51-year-old man with hand pain since striking a fence and sustaining a fifth metacarpal fracture. The patient in (*B*) is a 48-year-old woman with ulnar wrist pain and evidence of distal radioulnar joint instability.

plane.[17,25] As previously noted, the RSL attaches to the palmar aspect of the distal scaphoid pole and the central palmar capitate, whereas the LRL inserts widely on the palmar lunate (**Fig. 10**).[25] The RSL measures approximately 7.0 mm by 2.8 mm and the LRL 8.0 mm by 3.1 mm in the sagittal plane.[25]

Short radiolunate ligament Most commonly, the SRL appears as a homogeneously low-signal-intensity focal thickening of the joint capsule between the volar lip of the lunate facet and the volar lunate cortex (**Fig. 11**).[17] A study using MRA in cadaveric wrists more than a decade ago reported that the SRL was not well seen on MR imaging.[25]

Arcuate ligament The SCL, or radial limb of the arcuate ligament, and THL, or ulnar limb, appear as low-signal-intensity bands, often with intermediate signal striations, on all magnetic resonance sequences (**Fig. 12**).[17,20] The SCL arises from the scaphoid tuberosity, in common with the fibrous band of the RSL, and courses in a distal ulnar oblique fashion, 60 to the horizontal, deep to the RSL, to attach to the volar capitate body (**Fig. 13**).[20,25] The THL is seen to originate from the volar triquetrum and courses 30 from the horizontal in a distal-radial oblique fashion to attach to the volar capitate. A minority of patients in one series had secondary fibers from the THL attaching to the hamate as well.[20] These oblique ligaments may be best evaluated using oblique planes prescribed or reformatted along the long axes of these structures.[20] The SCL measures approximately 7.3 mm by 2.6 mm, and the THL 6.3 mm by 2.4 mm in the sagittal plane.[25]

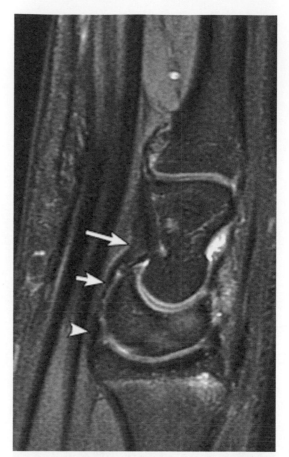

Fig. 11. Normal SRL. Sagittal T2-weighted fat-saturated image shows low-signal SRL (*arrowhead*) passing from the volar lip of the distal radius at the lunate facet, to the volar lunate cortex. Immediately distal to the SRL is the LRL (*short arrow*), followed by the distal RSL, near its capitate attachment (*arrow*). The patient is a 15-year-old female avid weight lifter with sudden-onset radial wrist pain during a clean-and-jerk maneuver.

Ulnocarpal ligaments Both the UTL and ULL are short, thick, low-signal-intensity structures on MR imaging, arising from the volar radioulnar ligament (**Fig. 14**).[17,25] The UTL has a visible broad insertion on the volar aspect of the triquetrum, and the ULL inserts on the volar aspect of the lunate, in common with the LRL.[25] The UTL measures approximately 5.8 mm by 3.0 mm, and the ULL 5.4 mm by 2.6 mm in the axial plane.[25] The MR imaging appearance of the UCL has yet to be reported.

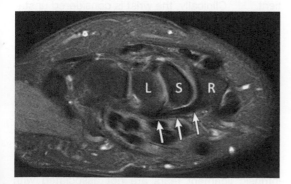

Fig. 10. Normal LRL in the same patient as in **Fig. 5**. Oblique axial T2-weighted fat-saturated image along the long axis of the LRL (*arrows*). Note the normal low signal intensity and thickness of this ligament as it passes from the radial styloid process (R), over the scaphoid (S), and to the volar lunate (L), deep to the carpal tunnel contents.

Dorsal capsular ligaments
Similar to the volar ligaments, the dorsal capsular ligaments also generally appear on MR imaging as linear hypointense structures,[25] often with alternating bands of intermediate signal intensity

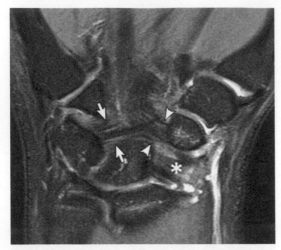

Fig. 12. Normal arcuate ligament. Coronal T2-weighted fat-saturated image shows normal, predominantly low-signal, striated radial (*arrowheads*) and ulnar (*arrows*) limbs of the arcuate ligament, or scaphocapitate (*arrowheads*) and triquetrohamocapitate (*arrows*) ligaments, respectively. The LRL (*asterisk*) is also seen with an associated multilobular ganglion cyst at its radial styloid origin. Same patient as **Fig. 11.**

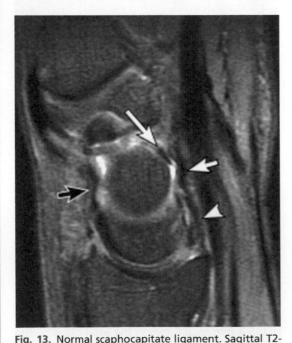

Fig. 13. Normal scaphocapitate ligament. Sagittal T2-weighted fat-saturated image at the radial margin of the capitate shows low-signal SCL (*long arrow*), or radial limb of arcuate ligament, in cross section, deep to the RSL (*white short arrow*). The normal LRL (*arrowhead*) and DIL (*black short arrow*) are also shown. The patient is a 43-year-old woman with wrist pain since a fall 3 months earlier, and who sustained a distal radius fracture 1 year earlier.

leading to a striated appearance.[17,19,21,23] In general, they are optimally evaluated in the axial and sagittal planes.[17,25] A recent study showed that the entire lengths of both DRL and DIL were seen in 80% of cases using 3 T MR imaging, and portions of both ligaments in 100% of cases.[66] Again, oblique axial reformats along the long axes of the ligaments were thought to best exhibit them.[66]

Dorsal radiocarpal ligament The DRL is usually seen arising near the Lister tubercle, extending over the dorsal lunate, and inserting on the triquetrum, proximal to the dorsal ridge (**Fig. 15**).[17,25,66] It measures approximately 5.5 mm by 1.7 mm in the sagittal plane.[25]

Dorsal intercarpal ligament Multiple variants of the DIL have been described, 4 of them on MR imaging.[23] The scaphotriquetral component of the DIL seems to be the most consistently visualized on MR imaging, with a trapezial branch, or fascicle, being less commonly identified with confidence.[25,66] It measures approximately 7.4 mm by 1.6 mm in the sagittal plane, and arises from the dorsal scaphoid, extending over the dorsal capitate, sending a thin, wide band of fibers to the dorsal lunate, and ultimately inserts on the triquetrum distal to the dorsal ridge (**Fig. 15**).[25,66]

PATHOLOGY

Ligamentous disorders, whether posttraumatic, congenital, degenerative, or some combination, can result in chronic pain in a stable wrist, and/or lead to carpal instability.[10,12,13] Carpal instability refers to a modification of the normal relationship between carpal bones in a symptomatic patient.[96–98] Clinically, the wrist is considered unstable if it shows symptomatic dysfunction, is not able to bear loads, and does not show normal kinematics during any portion of the wrist's arc of motion.[99,100] Radiologically, instability has traditionally been defined by loss of normal bone alignment either at rest, termed static instability, or during active motion, termed dynamic instability.[43,101,102] Both intrinsic ligaments, referred to as primary stabilizers, and extrinsic ligaments, referred to as secondary stabilizers, are important for maintaining carpal stability.[6,18,103,104] Isolated intrinsic ligament tears are not associated with carpal instability.[6] As in other parts of the body, imaging evidence of disorder must be carefully correlated with the patient's symptoms; in a recent study, an average of 3.15 abnormalities, including ligament tears, per asymptomatic wrist were identified on MR imaging.[105]

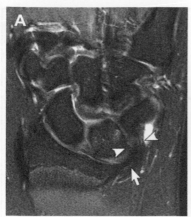
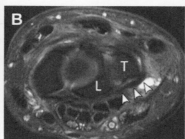
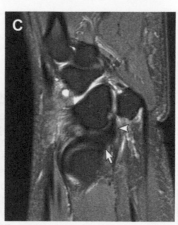

Fig. 14. Normal ulnocarpal ligaments. Coronal (*A*), axial (*B*), and sagittal (*C*) T2-weighted fat-saturated images show the normal low-signal collagenous sheet that comprises the ulnotriquetral and ulnolunate ligaments (*arrowheads*). Note the origin from the volar radioulnar ligament (*arrow*). The patient in (*A*) is a 14-year-old girl with hand pain. The patient in (*B*) and (*C*) is a 47-year-old woman with dorsoradial hand and wrist pain since a motor vehicle accident 1 day earlier. L, lunate; T, triquetrum.

Interosseous Ligaments

A tear that involves 1 or 2 of the 3 segments (volar, proximal, or dorsal) of either the SLL or LTL is considered a partial tear, whereas a tear of all 3 segments is a complete tear.[6,44,106] Note that this is different from a partial-thickness or full-thickness tear, also known as noncommunicating or communicating defects, respectively.[4,6] Partial tears with dynamic instability correspond with arthroscopic Geissler grades I and II, with a scapholunate gap of up to 3 mm on radiography.[2]

Grade III and IV lesions represent partial and complete SLL or LTL tears, with greater degrees of carpal instability, caused by additional compromised secondary stabilizers (**Table 1**).[2,104] Radiologists should note that this widely accepted arthroscopic grading scale quantifies carpal instability, rather than the extent or size of the SLL or LTL tear.[104] It is not complete interosseous ligament tears that cause instability, but rather a combination of interosseous ligament tear, which may be partial, such as the dorsal SLL, coupled with compromised secondary stabilizers or extrinsic ligament

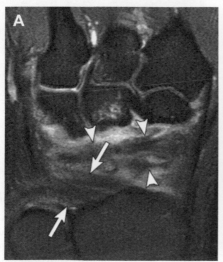
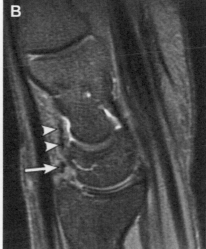

Fig. 15. Normal dorsal capsular ligaments. Coronal (*A*) and sagittal (*B*) T2-weighted fat-saturated images show low-signal DRL (*arrows*) and bifascicular (in these cases) DIL (*arrowheads*). The patient in (*A*) is a 31-year-old male construction worker who sustained a scaphoid fracture after a 6-m (20-foot) fall. The patient in (*B*) is the same patient as **Fig. 13**.

Table 1
Arthroscopic grading of interosseous ligament tears

Grade	—	Description	Radiographic Findings	
			Static Frontal View	Scapholunate Angle
I	Partial tear	Attenuation or hemorrhage of ligament as seen from radiocarpal joint Loss of smooth concave appearance between carpal bones	No gap	Normal
II	Partial tear	Incongruency or step-off seen from midcarpal joint space May be slight gap less than width of probe	Gap of 2–3 mm	50 –55
III	Partial or complete tear	Incongruency or step-off seen from midcarpal and radiocarpal joints Probe, but not 2.7-mm arthroscope, can be passed through gap	Gap of 3–5 mm	50 –60
IV	Complete tear	Incongruency or step-off seen from midcarpal and radiocarpal joints 2.7-mm arthroscope can be passed through gap. Gross instability	Gap of 5–6 mm	75 –80

tears.[6,8,63,107] Even a complete interosseous ligament tear could receive a low Geissler grade if the secondary stabilizers remain intact, preventing carpal instability.[6,63]

A tear can be confidently diagnosed when the ligament segment is absent or there is a fluid-filled discontinuity (**Figs. 16–19**).[6,7,12] Distortion of ligament morphology, including fraying, thinning or thickening, and irregularity; elongation or

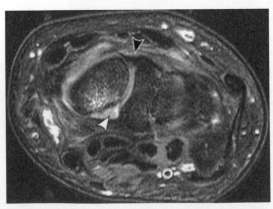

Fig. 16. Volar SLL tear. Axial T2-weighted fat-saturated images show an absence of the normal volar segment (*white arrowhead*), corresponding with this arthroscopic Geissler grade II tear, with adjacent scaphoid contusion. Note the normal, intact, triangular, low-signal dorsal SLL (*black arrowhead*). Same patient as **Fig. 11.**

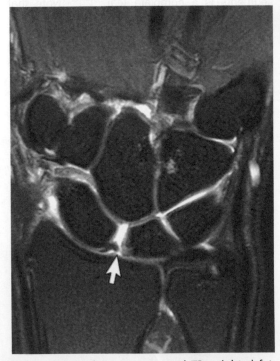

Fig. 17. Proximal SLL tear. Coronal T2-weighted fat-saturated image shows lunate detachment of the proximal segment (*arrow*) with scapholunate diastasis, corresponding with an arthroscopic Geissler grade III tear. The patient is a 37-year-old man who felt a pop and instant pain in the wrist after falling off a jet ski, with a positive Watson test.

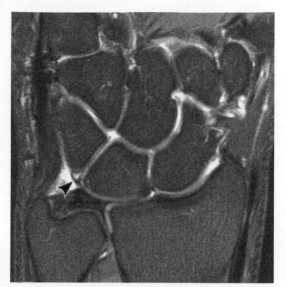

Fig. 18. Proximal lunotriquetral ligament tear. Coronal T2-weighted fat-saturated image shows abnormal fluid-signal intensity in the proximal segment (*arrowhead*) corresponding with this arthroscopic Geissler grade II tear. The patient is a 36-year-old man with chronic ulnar wrist pain since a fall on an outstretched hand 6 years earlier.

stretching; focal T2 hyperintensity or fluidlike signal; and abnormal ligament course, have all been reported as evidence for tear as well (**Figs. 20** and **21**).[7,12,44,106] However, these other

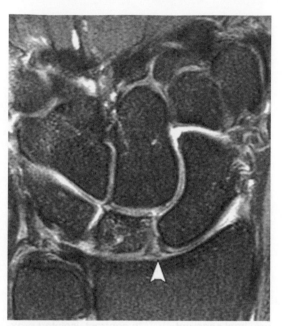

Fig. 20. Proximal SLL tear. Coronal T2-weighted fat-saturated image shows linear intrasubstance hyperintense signal through the full thickness of the membranous scapholunate segment (*arrowhead*), corresponding with an arthroscopic Geissler grade III tear. Same patient as **Fig. 9A**.

findings may overlap with asymptomatic degenerative changes, and therefore using them to diagnose tears may increase sensitivity at the cost of reduced specificity, depending on where along the receiver operating characteristic curve the clinician chooses to operate.[76,108] Specific secondary MR imaging findings that correlate with a

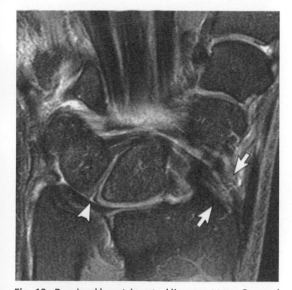

Fig. 19. Proximal lunotriquetral ligament tear. Coronal T2-weighted fat-saturated image shows abnormal linear fluid-signal intensity in the proximal segment (*arrowhead*) corresponding with this arthroscopic Geissler grade III tear. Also note the common origin of the RSL and LRL on the volar radial styloid process (*arrows*). Same patient as **Fig. 9A**.

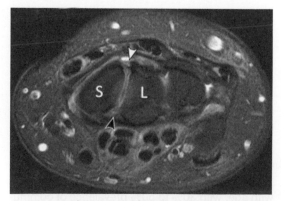

Fig. 21. Dorsal SLL tear in the same patient as in **Fig. 5**. Axial T2-weighted fat-saturated image shows abnormal linear T2 hyperintensity through the dorsal component (*white arrowhead*) with adjacent ganglion cyst, consistent with tear. Note the normal intermediate-signal-intensity volar segment (*black arrowhead*). S, scaphoid; L, lunate.

tear include widening of the intercarpal space or split-cartilage sign, focal osseous offset or incongruous joint, arc disruption, associated ganglion cyst, or focal chondromalacia/osteoarthritis (**Fig. 21**).[12,44,106] However, these secondary signs often have poor interobserver consistency and low sensitivity.[106]

Scapholunate ligament

SLL injury can occur with a fall on an outstretched hand in hyperextension, ulnar deviation, and internal supination, as part of Mayfield perilunar instability progression, associated with a concomitant injury such as distal-radial fracture, or as an isolated injury.[98,109,110] Patients often present with pain, swelling, and tenderness over the dorsoradial aspect of the wrist (see **Figs. 16, 17, 20** and **21**).[44] The volar, and particularly dorsal, segments of SLL are important for carpal stability.[6,8,63,107] Isolated dorsal or volar tears are unusual, probably because such tears quickly propagate into the proximal segment.[31,111] In contrast, isolated proximal segment defects are common and do not cause carpal instability.[31,107,112,113] Multiple arthrographic studies have shown that such defects commonly occur within both SLL and LTL as senescent changes in asymptomatic wrists.[114–118] Rarely present before 20 years of age,[46] half of all adults have SLL communicating defects by the age of 70 years, and 65% to 70% of those are bilateral.[112,113] However, not all proximal defects are asymptomatic; they can sometimes generate pain and do respond to surgical debridement.[10,11] It has also been reported that severe stretching of the SLL can occur, to the point that it is functionally incompetent, but without a perforation or frank tear.[44,98,110]

Lunotriquetral ligament

LTL injury may occur with a fall on an outstretched hand in maximal extension, radial deviation, and internal pronation, indicating reverse perilunar instability, as part of the later stages of perilunar instability, or as part of ulnocarpal abutment or impaction syndrome.[110,119,120] Patients often present with ulnar-sided wrist pain (**Figs. 18** and **19**).[44,120] The dorsal and particularly volar segments are important for carpal stability.[6,8] As in the SLL, isolated asymptomatic proximal defects are common,[114–118] often bilateral,[12] and increase with age, with 30% to 50% prevalence of communicating LTL defects in patients older than 50 years.[112,113] Volar and dorsal tears are nearly always associated with proximal segment tears, as in the SLL.[31,111] Even when the LTL is completely torn, lunotriquetral intercarpal joint widening is not typical, although arc disruption

may be seen.[17,44] LTL tears should be carefully assessed if there is a TFCC disorder, given the known high association (**Fig. 22**).[121]

Capsular Ligaments

The 2 most common categories of carpal instability are carpal instability dissociative (CID) and carpal instability nondissociative (CIND).[43,100,122] CID refers to loss of synchronous movement within the same carpal row, most commonly scapholunate dissociation, resulting in dorsal intercalated segmental instability (DISI) and lunotriquetral dissociation, resulting in volar intercalated segmental instability (VISI).[43,100,104] A DISI deformity consists of an abnormally flexed scaphoid and extended lunate caused by disruption of SLL and its secondary stabilizers, whereas a VISI deformity consists of a flexed lunate and extended triquetrum, caused by a disruption of LTL and its secondary stabilizers.[104] The specific roles of individual secondary stabilizers, or extrinsic ligaments, are still being worked out.

As in capsular ligaments elsewhere in the body, such as the medial collateral ligament of the knee,[123] wrist capsular ligament injury can have 3 progressive grades (**Box 2**).[4,6,17,28]

Radiocarpal and dorsal intercarpal ligaments

Capsular ligaments generally heal rapidly,[6,53] reconstituting with low-signal scar or fibrous tissue

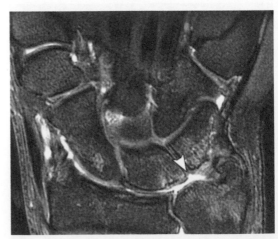

Fig. 22. Proximal lunotriquetral ligament tear in the setting of ulnocarpal impaction syndrome. Coronal T2-weighted fat-saturated image shows absence of normal proximal segment (*arrowhead*). Also note the large triangular fibrocartilage defect, ulna plus variance, and ulnar lunate cartilage loss with bony remodeling, which indicate ulnocarpal impaction syndrome. The patient is a 47-year-old man with chronic ulnar wrist pain that began insidiously and progressively worsened.

Box 2
Grades of ligamentous injury

I. Sprain: periligamentous edema and/or increased intrasubstance signal.

II. Partial tear: focal fluidlike signal intensity involving a portion of the cross section of the ligament; or abnormal morphologic features such as fraying, irregularity, indistinctness, or abnormal caliber.

III. Full-thickness tear: focal fluidlike signal or discontinuity extending across the entire ligament cross section.

that may appear similar to native ligament on MR imaging.[19,34] In these cases, diagnosis may be difficult, and comparison with known normal ligament measurements as described earlier,[6] or comparison with the contralateral wrist, may be helpful.[24] Persistence of carpal ligament defects may serve as proof of instability.[6,53]

According to a recent MR imaging study, the most frequently injured extrinsic ligaments are the RSL, LRL, and DRL (Figs. 23–27).[4] The RSL and LRL are often injured concomitantly (see Fig. 23).[34] Although injury to the radiocarpal ligaments are in general difficult to see on arthroscopy, because of wrist traction and poor visualization of osseous attachments,[2] dorsal capsular ligament tears are often even more challenging to directly visualize through the standard dorsal wrist arthroscopy portals, and volar wrist portals are not commonly used.[104] DRL tears

have been linked to the development of VISI, DISI, and even midcarpal instability,[57,61,62] and some clinicians advocate arthroscopic repair, even when torn in isolation.[104] The DIL plays an important role in stabilizing the scaphoid and preventing rotatory subluxation of the scaphoid following SLL disruption by acting as a tether.[60] Although the DIL was the most frequently completely torn extrinsic ligament in one series of patients with wrist trauma,[4] it was frequently, but only partially, torn in another series of patients with triquetral fractures (Figs. 28 and 29).[66]

The DRL and DIL together can be thought of as an indirect dorsal radioscaphoid ligament by way of the triquetrum (see Figs. 4 and 15A),[104] and may represent a teleologic compromise to

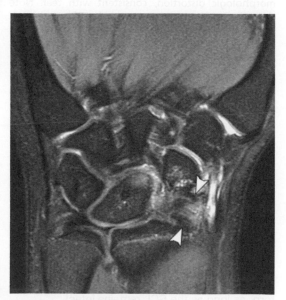

Fig. 23. Volar capsular ligament sprain. Coronal T2-weighted fat-saturated image shows hyperintense signal and thickening of the common origin of the RSL and LRL (arrowheads) consistent with grade I injury or sprain. Same patient as Fig. 11.

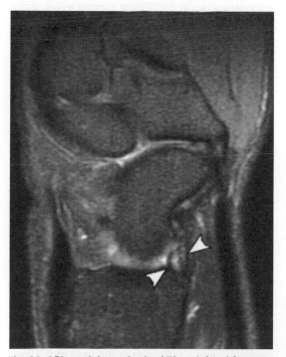

Fig. 24. LRL partial tear. Sagittal T2-weighted fat-saturated image shows markedly thickening proximal LRL (arrowheads) with hyperintense signal approaching fluid intensity consistent with grade II injury. Same patient as Fig. 13.

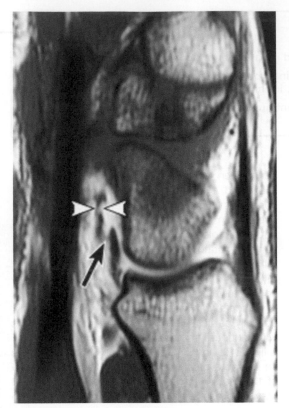

Fig. 25. RSL split tear. Sagittal T1-weighted image, with intra-articular gadolinium contrast agent, shows a full-thickness defect in the RSL (*arrowheads*), not to be confused with the normal interligamentous sulcus (*arrow*). The patient is a 24-year-old man who sustained a trapezoid fracture after punching another person.

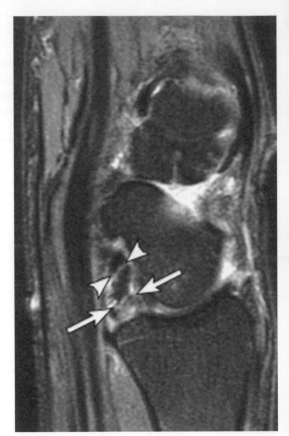

Fig. 26. LRL split tear. Sagittal T2-weighted fat-saturated image shows linear hyperintense signal through the LRL (*arrows*) with associated thickening and morphologic distortion, consistent with tear. Note the adjacent interligamentous sulcus (*arrowheads*). The patient is a 54-year-old woman with injury to the upper extremity from a motor vehicle accident 2 weeks earlier.

preserve range of motion while maintaining stability.[65] Cadaveric sectioning studies indicate that disruption of both dorsal SLL and the scaphoid attachment of DIL are required for dynamic scapholunate diastasis and rotatory instability of the scaphoid, but an additional disruption of either the lunate attachment of DIL or DRL is required to cause DISI.[60,63]

Volar midcarpal ligaments

CIND refers to loss of synchronous motion between carpal rows or between the distal radius and proximal carpal row. The most common subtype of CIND is known as palmar midcarpal instability (PMCI), characterized by a painful sudden clunking of the wrist with axial loading and ulnar deviation, and a volar sag at the level of the midcarpal joint.[124] It is caused by failure or laxity of palmar midcarpal ligaments, such as the arcuate ligament, and a VISI pattern may or may not be seen.[104,124] Although PMCI greatly impairs

activities of daily living, primarily because of decreased range of radial and ulnar deviation, patients often report no trauma history or only a minor injury.[125] If conservative therapy fails, surgery with soft tissue reconstruction or arthrodesis is considered.[124] There are anecdotal reports of discrete tears of the arcuate ligament, as well as a stretched or redundant appearance, in patients with PMCI, but this has yet to be proved.[126]

STL injury on MR imaging is also not well described, being inferred on arthrography via abnormal extension of contrast into the flexor carpi radialis tendon sheath.[42] The scaphotrapeziotrapezoid joint may seem normal even if the STL is torn, as long as the SCL remains intact.[42]

Ulnocarpal ligaments

Partial tears of the UTL are common, often resulting in a longitudinal split and presenting with

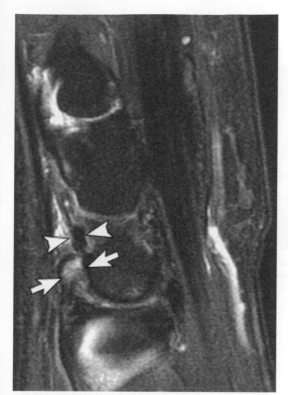

Fig. 27. DRL partial tear. Sagittal T2-weighted fat-saturated image shows marked hyperintense signal with moderate thickening of the distal DRL (*arrows*) near its triquetral attachment. Note the nearby normal low-signal DIL (*arrowheads*). The patient is a 36-year-old man with dorsal wrist pain since a fall while playing softball.

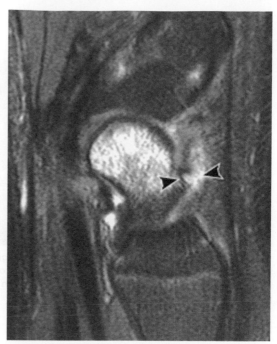

Fig. 29. DIL tear. Sagittal T2-weighted, fat-saturated image shows interruption of the scaphoid attachment of the DIL with fluid-signal (*arrowheads*), consistent with a high-grade partial tear. Note the scaphoid hyperintense signal caused by osseous hemorrhage and edema from scaphoid fracture evident on a separate image. The patient is a 16-year-old boy who fell off a skateboard and sustained a distal scaphoid fracture.

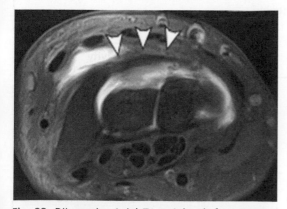

Fig. 28. DIL sprain. Axial T1-weighted, fat-saturated image with intra-articular gadolinium contrast agent shows marked thickening and fraying of the DIL (*arrowheads*), which is a common imaging correlate to the dorsal capsular wrist sprain. The patient is a 37-year-old man with dorsal wrist pain and instability after falling a few days earlier.

chronic ulnar-sided wrist pain that worsens with gripping, which may or may not have been preceded by a traumatic event.[127] A fluid-filled discontinuity is uncommonly seen; however, localizing abnormal T2 hyperintensity in the UTL, especially when using a microscopy coil, often correlates with arthroscopic evidence of partial UTL split tear (**Fig. 30**).[17,59] The presence of ulnar fovea tenderness, or positive ulnar fovea sign, in the stable wrist is typical in these patients.[127,128] Although the disorder is typically directly viewed from the 3-4 portal, distal triquetral attachment site abnormalities often cannot be directly seen arthroscopically.[59,127] Surgical repair has good outcomes with essentially no complications.[127]

Complete ulnocarpal ligament tear, or foveal dissociation, results in distal radioulnar joint instability.[127] On MR imaging, a fluid-filled discontinuity either at the triquetral attachment of the UTL or at the foveal attachment may be seen, with resultant ligamentous retraction and laxity.[17] MR imaging findings for UCL tears have yet to be reported.

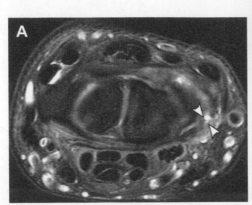
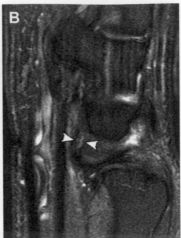

Fig. 30. Ulnotriquetral ligament tear. Axial (*A*) and sagittal (*B*) T2-weighted, fat-saturated images show linear T2 prolongation in the distal ulnotriquetral ligament (*arrowheads*), consistent with arthroscopically proven longitudinal split tear. The patient is a 44-year-old man with insidious-onset chronic ulnar wrist pain, exacerbated by playing tennis.

DIAGNOSTIC PERFORMANCE OF MR IMAGING
Scapholunate and Lunotriquetral Ligaments

A meta-analysis of the major diagnostic performance studies preceding the year 2000[7,21,28,29,73,129] concluded that MR imaging had an overall adjusted sensitivity/specificity of 70%/90% for SLL tears, and 56%/91% for LTL tears, compared with arthroscopy.[26] Field strengths from 0.5 T to 1.5 T were included in the analysis, and higher sensitivity and accuracy was achieved whenever T2*-weighted 3D GRE sequences were used, probably because of the thinner slices and higher spatial resolution achievable with this technique.[26] Diagnostic performance studies published since then have generally shown further improved specificity, at or approaching 100% for both SLL and LTL tears at 3 T,[30,33,130,131] or at 1.5 T with intra-articular

Table 2
Diagnostic performance of noncontrast wrist MR imaging

Reference, Year	No. of Wrists	Field Strength (T)	Partial Tears Included?	SLL Sensitivity (%)	SLL Specificity (%)	LTL Sensitivity (%)	LTL Specificity (%)
Haims et al,[72] 2003	45	1.5	Complete	41	90	40	92
Moser et al,[32] 2007[a]	45	1.5	Partial	59–77	70–83	30–50	94–97
Anderson et al,[33] 2008	70	1.5	Complete	57	83	22	94
Anderson et al,[33] 2008	32	3	Complete	70	94	50	94
Magee,[30] 2009	49	3	Complete	89	100	82	100
Lee et al,[130] 2013[b]	48	3	Complete	65	100	62	100
Spaans et al,[131] 2013	38	3	Partial	70–81	100	NA	NA
Srivastava et al,[36] 2014	16	1.5	Partial	62	100	40	100

Abbreviation: NA, not available.
[a] Clinical follow-up was also used as reference standard in addition to arthroscopy in this study.
[b] No axial images were evaluated on the noncontrast images.

Table 3
Diagnostic performance wrist MRA

Reference, Year	No. of Wrists	Field Strength (T)	Partial Tears Included?	SLL Sensitivity (%)	SLL Specificity (%)	LTL Sensitivity (%)	LTL Specificity (%)
Manton et al,[106] 2001[a]	17	1.5	Partial	56	56	31	76
Schmitt et al,[132] 2003[b]	125	1.5	Complete	92	100	NA	NA
			Partial	62	100	NA	NA
Moser et al,[32] 2007	45	1.5	Partial	68–77	87	50–60	94–97
Magee,[30] 2009	35	3	Complete	100	100	100	100
Mahmood et al,[35] 2012	30	1.5	?	91	88	100	100
Lee et al, 2013	48	3	Complete	85	97	85	100
Srivastava et al,[36] 2014	16	1.5	Partial	100	100	100	100

Abbreviation: NA, not available.

[a] Indirect arthrography was performed via intravenous injection of 20 mL of gadopentetate dimeglumine rather than intra-articular gadolinium in this study and only coronal plane images were evaluated.

[b] No axial images were evaluated.

gadolinium (**Tables 2** and **3**).[32,35,36,132] The 1 study that had unusually low specificity was the only study that used indirect arthrography via an intravenous injection rather than an intra-articular injection.[106]

In contrast, sensitivity has not significantly improved in more recent noncontrast MR imaging studies, even at 3 T, with sensitivities ranging from 41% to 89% for SLL tears and 22% to 82% for LTL tears, although these studies more commonly include partial tears, making direct comparison difficult (**Table 2**).[30,32,33,36,72,130,131] One study that directly compared 1.5 T with 3 T found a statistically insignificant increase in sensitivity for both SLL and LTL tears.[33] Studies including MRA generally report higher sensitivity: 62% to 100% for SLL tears and 50% to 100% for LTL tears (**Table 3**).[30,32,35,36,130,132] Articles that directly compared noncontrast MR imaging with MRA generally showed improved sensitivity for both SLL and LTL tears as well using intra-articular gadolinium.[30,32,36,130] There is substantial interobserver agreement with both noncontrast MR imaging and MRA for diagnosing interosseous ligament tears.[6,32]

Sensitivity for partial tears is reportedly lower than for complete tears: 62% for partial SLL tears compared with 92% for complete tears in one study,[132] and 47% to 71% compared with 100% in another study,[32] both at 1.5 T. MRA increased sensitivity for partial SLL tears from 47–71% to 59–71% and LTL tears from 22–44% to 44–56% in one study.[32] Specificity for partial tears may still be as high as 100%.[132] Two cadaveric studies attempted to address diagnostic performance of specific interosseous ligament segments.[31,111] Schmid and colleagues[31] combined the segments of SLL and LTL, and calculated a sensitivity/specificity of 0%/100%, 79%/25%, and 60%/77% for dorsal, proximal, and volar segment tears, respectively, in 9 cadaveric wrists at 1.5 T, but with poor interobserver agreement. Lee and colleagues[111] showed improved sensitivity for individual SLL segment tears (partial tears) from 50% to 66% using noncontrast MR imaging to 100% with MRA, and fairly stable specificity at 86% to 100%. The proximal LTL segment sensitivity improved from 60% to 100% with MRA, but the dorsal and volar LTL segments remained at 50% sensitivity.[111] Specificity for LTL segment tears (partial tears) was 89% to 100% with noncontrast MR imaging and 100% for all 3 segments with MRA.[111]

Conclusion and caveats

Modern optimized noncontrast MR imaging, especially at 3 T, has excellent specificity and good sensitivity for SLL and LTL tears.[26,30,33,130,131] Therefore, MR imaging of interosseous ligaments is a test with a very high positive likelihood ratio, and a moderately low negative likelihood ratio. Such a test is expected to be more useful when positive, because it is ideal for ruling in disorders rather than ruling them out.[133] The use of MRA may increase sensitivity, which would decrease the negative likelihood ratio, making MR imaging a better screening test, but at the expense of no longer being completely noninvasive.[28,30,32,36,77,81,83,130] MR imaging, including MRA, remains less invasive, safer, and less expensive than diagnostic arthroscopy.[14,134]

It should be emphasized that the numbers reported earlier are estimates of the true sensitivity and specificity of wrist MR imaging. Because most patients with negative MR imaging examinations do not go on to arthroscopy, and arthroscopy cannot be ethically performed on normal volunteers, there is a large bias of overly prevalent ligament disorders in the patient populations studied in the literature.[30,32,131] Compounded by the retrospective design of many available diagnostic performance studies, the small sample sizes used, and the known error rate of the arthroscopy reference standard, the stated estimates of MR imaging accuracy, particularly specificity, should be understood to have wide confidence intervals.[26,32] In addition, the expertise and experience of the interpreting radiologist is likely to affect not only accuracy but resultant clinical management.[17,33,134]

Capsular Ligaments

In contrast with the interosseous ligaments of the proximal carpal row, extrinsic ligament tears have rarely been studied. One major difficulty is the lack of a reliable reference standard.[6,34] As previously described, evaluation of the extrinsic ligaments using arthroscopy is incomplete at best, particularly near osseous attachments, and in general with traction applied.[2,6,34,50,59] Despite this shortcoming, several studies have attempted to assess the diagnostic performance of MR imaging for certain extrinsic ligaments using arthroscopy as a reference standard.[7,21,27,28,33,34,59] Scheck and colleagues[28] calculated a sensitivity/specificity of 67%/88%, and 50%/100% for noncontrast 1.5 T MR imaging of complete RSL and LRL tears, respectively, which improved to 100%/100% and 100%/94% with MRA. More recently, Mak and colleagues[34] included partial tears, and found a lower sensitivity/specificity of RSL and LTL tears: 63%/56% and 25%/68%, respectively, with MRA at 1.5 T.

Ulnocarpal ligament (UTL/ULL) tear sensitivity/specificity has been reported as 57%/89% at 1.5 T,[33] 67%/87% at 3 T,[33] and 100%/70% using a microscopy coil.[59] The sensitivity/specificity for a specific type of UTL tear, known as a longitudinal split tear,[127] was 58%/60% by one reader in one study at 3 T.[27] Further study is required before

any meaningful conclusions can be made regarding the performance of MR imaging for capsular ligament disorders. Given arthroscopy's shortcomings as a reference standard, alternatives need to be considered. For example, Theumann and colleagues[6] used radiographic evidence of carpal instability as indirect evidence of coexisting extrinsic and intrinsic ligament disorders in a group of patients in whom all 22 extrinsic ligament tears seen on MR imaging were missed on arthroscopy, possibly because of the location of tears at bony attachments. In addition, larger prospective and sufficiently powered imaging studies are needed.[34]

SUMMARY

Modern MR imaging using currently available surface coils and pulse sequences can readily and consistently visualize all of the major wrist ligaments involved in pathology. Specificity for complete and partial SLL and LTL tears is excellent, whereas sensitivity is good for complete tears and moderate for partial tears. The use of higher field strengths, thinner and oblique slices, and MRA improve sensitivity for both partial and complete tears, making MR imaging a better noninvasive screening test. Radiologists, who are aware of the anatomy, routinely visualize the extrinsic and capsular ligaments, although further study of their disorders and diagnostic performance is required.

REFERENCES

1. Caloia MF, Gallino RN, Caloia H, et al. Incidence of ligamentous and other injuries associated with scaphoid fractures during arthroscopically assisted reduction and percutaneous fixation. Arthroscopy 2008;24(7):754–9.
2. Geissler WB, Freeland AE, Savoie FH, et al. Intracarpal soft-tissue lesions associated with an intra-articular fracture of the distal end of the radius. J Bone Joint Surg Am 1996;78(3):357–65.
3. Jørgsholm P, Thomsen NO, Björkman A, et al. The incidence of intrinsic and extrinsic ligament injuries in scaphoid waist fractures. J Hand Surg Am 2010; 35(3):368–74.
4. Taneja AK, Bredella MA, Chang CY, et al. Extrinsic wrist ligaments: prevalence of injury by magnetic resonance imaging and association with intrinsic ligament tears. J Comput Assist Tomogr 2013; 37(5):783–9.
5. Larsen CF, Lauritsen J. Epidemiology of acute wrist trauma. Int J Epidemiol 1993;22(5):911–6.
6. Theumann NH, Etechami G, Duvoisin B, et al. Association between extrinsic and intrinsic carpal ligament injuries at MR arthrography and carpal

instability at radiography: initial observations 1. Radiology 2006;238(3):950–7.

7. Zlatkin MB, Chao PC, Osterman AL, et al. Chronic wrist pain: evaluation with high-resolution MR imaging. Radiology 1989;173(3):723–9.

8. Timins ME, Jahnke JP, Krah SF, et al. MR imaging of the major carpal stabilizing ligaments: normal anatomy and clinical examples. Radiographics 1995;15(3):575–87.

9. Mikić ZD. Age changes in the triangular fibrocartilage of the wrist joint. J Anat 1978;126(Pt 2): 367–84.

10. Weiss AP, Sachar K, Glowacki KA. Arthroscopic debridement alone for intercarpal ligament tears. J Hand Surg Am 1997;22(2):344–9.

11. Ruch DS, Poehling GG. Arthroscopic management of partial scapholunate and lunotriquetral injuries of the wrist. J Hand Surg Am 1996;21(3):412–7.

12. Daunt N. Magnetic resonance imaging of the wrist: anatomy and pathology of interosseous ligaments and the triangular fibrocartilage complex. Curr Probl Diagn Radiol 2002;31(4):158–76.

13. Watson HK, Weinzweig J, Zeppieri J. The natural progression of scaphoid instability. Hand Clin 1997;13(1):39–49.

14. Hobby JL, Dixon AK, Bearcroft PW, et al. MR imaging of the wrist: effect on clinical diagnosis and patient care. Radiology 2001;220(3):589–93.

15. Nikken JJ, Oei EH, Ginai AZ, et al. Acute wrist trauma: value of a short dedicated extremity MR imaging examination in prediction of need for treatment 1. Radiology 2005;234(1):116–24.

16. American College of Radiology. ACR–SCBT-MR–SPR–SSR practice parameter for the performance of magnetic resonance imaging (MRI) of the wrist [Internet]. 2007. Available at: http://www.acr.org/~/media/ACR/Documents/PGTS/guidelines/MRI_Wrist.pdf. Accessed October 30, 2014.

17. Ringler MD. MRI of wrist ligaments. J Hand Surg Am 2013;38(10):2034–46.

18. Taljanovic M, Malan J, Sheppard J. Normal anatomy of the extrinsic capsular wrist ligaments by 3-T MRI and high-resolution ultrasonography. Semin Musculoskelet Radiol 2012;16(02):104–14.

19. Shahabpour M, De Maeseneer M, Pouders C, et al. MR imaging of normal extrinsic wrist ligaments using thin slices with clinical and surgical correlation. Eur J Radiol 2011;77(2):196–201.

20. Chang W, Peduto AJ, Aguiar RO, et al. Arcuate ligament of the wrist: normal MR appearance and its relationship to palmar midcarpal instability: a cadaveric study. Skeletal Radiol 2007; 36(7):641–5.

21. Totterman SM, Miller R, Wasserman B, et al. Intrinsic and extrinsic carpal ligaments: evaluation by three-dimensional Fourier transform MR imaging. AJR Am J Roentgenol 1993;160(1):117–23.

22. Totterman SM, Miller RJ. Scapholunate ligament: normal MR appearance on three-dimensional gradient-recalled-echo images. Radiology 1996; 200(1):237–41.

23. Smith DK. Dorsal carpal ligaments of the wrist: normal appearance on multiplanar reconstructions of three-dimensional Fourier transform MR imaging. AJR Am J Roentgenol 1993;161(1):119–25.

24. Smith DK. Volar carpal ligaments of the wrist: normal appearance on multiplanar reconstructions of three-dimensional Fourier transform MR imaging. AJR Am J Roentgenol 1993;161(2):353–7.

25. Theumann NH, Pfirrmann CW, Antonio GE, et al. Extrinsic carpal ligaments: normal MR arthrographic appearance in cadavers 1. Radiology 2003;226(1):171–9.

26. Hobby JL, Tom BD, Bearcroft PW, et al. Magnetic resonance imaging of the wrist: diagnostic performance statistics. Clin Radiol 2001;56(1):50–7.

27. Ringler MD, Howe BM, Amrami KK, et al. Utility of magnetic resonance imaging for detection of longitudinal split tear of the ulnotriquetral ligament. J Hand Surg Am 2013;38(9):1723–7.

28. Scheck RJ, Romagnolo A, Hierner R. The carpal ligaments in MR arthrography of the wrist: correlation with standard MRI and wrist arthroscopy. J Magn Reson Imaging 1999;9(3):468–74.

29. Potter HG, Asnis-Ernberg L, Weiland AJ, et al. The utility of high-resolution magnetic resonance imaging in the evaluation of the triangular fibrocartilage complex of the wrist. J Bone Joint Surg Am 1997; 79(11):1675–84.

30. Magee T. Comparison of 3-T MRI and arthroscopy of intrinsic wrist ligament and TFCC tears. AJR Am J Roentgenol 2009;192(1):80–5.

31. Schmid MR, Schertler T, Pfirrmann CW, et al. Interosseous ligament tears of the wrist: comparison of multi-detector row CT arthrography and MR imaging 1. Radiology 2005;237(3):1008–13.

32. Moser T, Dosch JC, Moussaoui A, et al. Wrist ligament tears: evaluation of MRI and combined MDCT and MR arthrography. AJR Am J Roentgenol 2007; 188(5):1278–86.

33. Anderson ML, Skinner JA, Felmlee JP, et al. Diagnostic comparison of 1.5 Tesla and 3.0 Tesla preoperative MRI of the wrist in patients with ulnar-sided wrist pain. J Hand Surg Am 2008; 33(7):1153–9.

34. Mak WH, Szabo RM, Myo GK. Assessment of volar radiocarpal ligaments: MR arthrographic and arthroscopic correlation. AJR Am J Roentgenol 2012;198(2):423–7.

35. Mahmood A. Wrist MRI arthrogram v wrist arthroscopy: what are we finding? Open Orthop J 2012; 6(1):194–8.

36. Srivastava D, Sharma R, Gamanagatti S, et al. Comparison of conventional MRI and MR

arthrography in the evaluation wrist ligament tears: a preliminary experience. Indian J Radiol Imaging 2014;24(3):259.

37. American College of Radiology. ACR appropriateness criteria: chronic wrist pain [Internet]. 1998. Available at: http://www.acr.org/~/media/ACR/Documents/AppCriteria/Diagnostic/ChronicWristPain.pdf. Accessed October 30, 2014.

38. Berger RA. The anatomy of the ligaments of the wrist and distal radioulnar joints. Clin Orthop Relat Res 2001;383:32–40.

39. Berger RA. The anatomy and basic biomechanics of the wrist joint. J Hand Ther 1996; 9(2):84–93.

40. Berger RA. The ligaments of the wrist. A current overview of anatomy with considerations of their potential functions. Hand Clin 1997;13(1):63–82.

41. Taleisnik J. The ligaments of the wrist. J Hand Surg Am 1976;1(2):110–8.

42. Bateni CP, Bartolotta RJ, Richardson ML, et al. Imaging key wrist ligaments: what the surgeon needs the radiologist to know. AJR Am J Roentgenol 2013;200(5):1089–95.

43. Taleisnik J. Current concepts review. Carpal instability. J Bone Joint Surg Am 1988;70(8):1262–8.

44. Zlatkin MB, Rosner J. MR imaging of ligaments and triangular fibrocartilage complex of the wrist. Magn Reson Imaging Clin North Am 2004;12(2): 301–31.

45. Berger RA. The gross and histologic anatomy of the scapholunate interosseous ligament. J Hand Surg Am 1996;21(2):170–8.

46. Viegas SF, Ballantyne DG. Attritional lesions of the wrist joint. J Hand Surg Am 1987;12(6):1025–9.

47. Berger RA, Imeada T, Berglund L, et al. Constraint and material properties of the subregions of the scapholunate interosseous ligament. J Hand Surg Am 1999;24(5):953–62.

48. Ritt MJ, Bishop AT, Berger RA, et al. Lunotriquetral ligament properties: a comparison of three anatomic subregions. J Hand Surg Am 1998; 23(3):425–31.

49. Shin AY, Battaglia MJ, Bishop AT. Lunotriquetral instability: diagnosis and treatment. J Am Acad Orthop Surg 2000;8(3):170–9.

50. Rominger MB, Bernreuter WK, Kenney PJ, et al. MR imaging of anatomy and tears of wrist ligaments. Radiographics 1993;13(6):1233–46 [discussion: 1247–8].

51. Rayhack JM, Linscheid RL, Dobyns JH, et al. Posttraumatic ulnar translation of the carpus. J Hand Surg Am 1987;12(2):180–9.

52. Adler BD, Logan PM, Janzen DL, et al. Extrinsic radiocarpal ligaments: magnetic resonance imaging of normal wrists and scapholunate dissociation. Can Assoc Radiol J 1996;47(6):417–22.

53. Berger RA, Landsmeer JM. The palmar radiocarpal ligaments: a study of adult and fetal human wrist joints. J Hand Surg Am 1990;15(6):847–54.

54. North ER, Thomas S. An anatomic guide for arthroscopic visualization of the wrist capsular ligaments. J Hand Surg Am 1988;13(6):815–22.

55. Mayfield JK, Johnson RP, Kilcoyne RF. The ligaments of the human wrist and their functional significance. Anat Rec 1976;186(3):417–28.

56. Berger RA, Blair WF. The radioscapholunate ligament: a gross and histologic description. Anat Rec 1984;210(2):393–405.

57. Viegas SF, Patterson RM, Peterson PD, et al. Ulnar-sided perilunate instability: an anatomic and biomechanic study. J Hand Surg Am 1990;15(2): 268–78.

58. Garcia-Elias M. Soft-tissue anatomy and relationships about the distal ulna. Hand Clin 1998;14(2): 165–76.

59. Tanaka T, Yoshioka H, Ueno T, et al. Comparison between high-resolution MRI with a microscopy coil and arthroscopy in triangular fibrocartilage complex injury. J Hand Surg Am 2006;31(8): 1308–14.

60. Elsaidi GA, Ruch DS, Kuzma GR, et al. Dorsal wrist ligament insertions stabilize the scapholunate interval: cadaver study. Clin Orthop Relat Res 2004; 425:152–7.

61. Horii E, Garcia-Elias M, An KN, et al. A kinematic study of luno-triquetral dissociations. J Hand Surg Am 1991;16(2):355–62.

62. Moritomo H, Viegas SF, Elder KW, et al. Scaphoid nonunions: a 3-dimensional analysis of patterns of deformity. J Hand Surg Am 2000;25(3):520–8.

63. Mitsuyasu H, Patterson RM, Shah MA, et al. The role of the dorsal intercarpal ligament in dynamic and static scapholunate instability. J Hand Surg Am 2004;29(2):279–88.

64. Osterman AL, Seidman GD. The role of arthroscopy in the treatment of lunatotriquetral ligament injuries. Hand Clin 1995;11(1):41–50.

65. Viegas SF, Yamaguchi S, Boyd NL, et al. The dorsal ligaments of the wrist: anatomy, mechanical properties, and function. J Hand Surg Am 1999;24(3): 456–68.

66. Becce F, Theumann N, Bollmann C, et al. Dorsal fractures of the triquetrum: MRI findings with an emphasis on dorsal carpal ligament injuries. AJR Am J Roentgenol 2013;200(3):608–17.

67. Mizuseki T, Ikuta Y. The dorsal carpal ligaments: their anatomy and function. J Hand Surg Br 1989; 14(1):91–8.

68. Steinbach LS, Smith DK. MRI of the wrist. Clin Imaging 2000;24(5):298–322.

69. Hricak H, Amparo EG. Body MRI: alleviation of claustrophobia by prone positioning. Radiology 1984;152(3):819.

70. Kulkarni MV, Patton JA, Price RR. Technical considerations for the use of surface coils in MRI. AJR Am J Roentgenol 1986;147(2):373–8.

71. Kocharian A, Adkins MC, Amrami KK, et al. Wrist: improved MR imaging with optimized transmit-receive coil design. Radiology 2002; 223(3):870–6.

72. Haims AH, Schweitzer ME, Morrison WB, et al. Internal derangement of the wrist: indirect MR arthrography versus unenhanced MR imaging 1. Radiology 2003;227(3):701–7.

73. Schweitzer ME, Brahme SK, Hodler J, et al. Chronic wrist pain: spin-echo and short tau inversion recovery MR imaging and conventional and MR arthrography. Radiology 1992;182(1):205–11.

74. Dick EA, Burnett C, Gedroyc WM. MRI of the wrist. Radiography 2008;14(3):246–54.

75. Morley J, Bidwell J, Bransby-Zachary M. A comparison of the findings of wrist arthroscopy and magnetic resonance imaging in the investigation of wrist pain. J Hand Surg Br 2001;26(6): 544–6.

76. Yoshioka H, Tanaka T, Ueno T, et al. High-resolution MR imaging of the proximal zone of the lunotriquetral ligament with a microscopy coil. Skeletal Radiol 2006;35(5):288–94.

77. Saupe N, Prüssmann KP, Luechinger R, et al. MR imaging of the wrist: comparison between 1.5- and 3-T MR imaging—preliminary experience 1. Radiology 2005;234(1):256–64.

78. Lenk S, Ludescher B, Martirosan P, et al. 3.0 T high-resolution MR imaging of carpal ligaments and TFCC. Rofo 2004;176(5):664–7.

79. Chang G, Friedrich KM, Wang L, et al. MRI of the wrist at 7 tesla using an eight-channel array coil combined with parallel imaging: preliminary results. J Magn Reson Imaging 2010;31(3):740–6.

80. Totterman SM, Miller RJ, McCance SE, et al. Lesions of the triangular fibrocartilage complex: MR findings with a three-dimensional gradient-recalled-echo sequence. Radiology 1996;199(1):227–32.

81. Scheck RJ, Kubitzek C, Hierner R, et al. The scapholunate interosseous ligament in MR arthrography of the wrist: correlation with non-enhanced MRI and wrist arthroscopy. Skeletal Radiol 1997; 26(5):263–71.

82. Smith DK. Scapholunate interosseous ligament of the wrist: MR appearances in asymptomatic volunteers and arthrographically normal wrists. Radiology 1994;192(1):217–21.

83. Zanetti M, Bräm J, Hodler J. Triangular fibrocartilage and intercarpal ligaments of the wrist: does MR arthrography improve standard MRI? J Magn Reson Imaging 1997;7(3):590–4.

84. Yu JS, Habib PA. Normal MR imaging anatomy of the wrist and hand. Radiol Clin North Am 2006; 44(4):569–81, viii.

85. Stevens KJ, Wallace CG, Chen W, et al. Imaging of the wrist at 1.5 tesla using isotropic three-dimensional fast spin echo cube. J Magn Reson Imaging 2011;33(4):908–15.

86. Robinson G, Chung T, Finlay K, et al. Axial oblique MR imaging of the intrinsic ligaments of the wrist: initial experience. Skeletal Radiol 2006;35(10): 765–73.

87. Rubin DA, Kneeland JB. MR imaging of the musculoskeletal system: technical considerations for enhancing image quality and diagnostic yield. AJR Am J Roentgenol 1994;163(5):1155–63.

88. Mirowitz SA. Fast scanning and fat-suppression MR imaging of musculoskeletal disorders. AJR Am J Roentgenol 1993;161(6):1147–57.

89. Maas M, Dijkstra PF, Akkerman EM. Uniform fat suppression in hands and feet through the use of two-point Dixon chemical shift MR imaging. Radiology 1999;210(1):189–93.

90. Fleckenstein JL, Archer BT, Barker BA, et al. Fast short-tau inversion-recovery MR imaging. Radiology 1991;179(2):499 504.

91. Bieri O, Scheffler K. Fundamentals of balanced steady state free precession MRI. J Magn Reson Imaging 2013;38(1):2–11.

92. Boutin RD, Buonocore MH, Immerman I, et al. Real-time magnetic resonance imaging (MRI) during active wrist motion—initial observations. PLoS One 2013;8(12):e84004.

93. Gheno R, Buck FM, Nico MA, et al. Differences between radial and ulnar deviation of the wrist in the study of the intrinsic intercarpal ligaments: magnetic resonance imaging and gross anatomic inspection in cadavers. Skeletal Radiol 2009;39(8): 799–805.

94. Burns JE, Tanaka T, Ueno T, et al. Pitfalls that may mimic injuries of the triangular fibrocartilage and proximal intrinsic wrist ligaments at MR imaging 1. Radiographics 2011;31(1):63–78.

95. Smith DK, Snearly WN. Lunotriquetral interosseous ligament of the wrist: MR appearances in asymptomatic volunteers and arthrographically normal wrists. Radiology 1994;191(1):199–202.

96. Gilula LA, Weeks PM. Post-traumatic ligamentous instabilities of the wrist 1. Radiology 1978;129(3): 641–51.

97. Linscheid RL, Dobyns JH, Beabout JW, et al. Traumatic instability of the wrist. Diagnosis, classification, and pathomechanics. J Bone Joint Surg Am 1972;54(8):1612–32.

98. Mayfield JK. Wrist ligamentous anatomy and pathogenesis of carpal instability. Orthop Clin North Am 1984;15(2):209–16.

99. Garcia-Elias M. Definition of carpal instability: the Anatomy and Biomechanics Committee of the International Federation of Societies for Surgery of the hand. J Hand Surg Am 1999;24(4):866–7.

100. Garcia-Elias M. The treatment of wrist instability. J Hand Surg Br 1997;79(4):684–90.

101. Schernberg F. Roentgenographic examination of the wrist: a systematic study of the normal, lax and injured wrist. Part 2: stress views. J Hand Surg Br 1990;15(2):220–8.

102. Watson HK, Ryu J, Akelman E. Limited triscaphoid intercarpal arthrodesis for rotatory subluxation of the scaphoid. J Bone Joint Surg Am 1986;68(3): 345–9.

103. Brown RR, Fliszar E, Cotten A, et al. Extrinsic and intrinsic ligaments of the wrist: normal and pathologic anatomy at MR arthrography with three-compartment enhancement. Radiographics 1998; 18(3):667–74.

104. Slutsky DJ. Incidence of dorsal radiocarpal ligament tears in the presence of other intercarpal derangements. Arthroscopy 2008;24(5):526–33.

105. Couzens G, Daunt N, Crawford R, et al. Positive magnetic resonance imaging findings in the asymptomatic wrist. ANZ J Surg 2014;84(7–8): 528–32.

106. Manton GL, Schweitzer ME, Weishaupt D, et al. Partial interosseous ligament tears of the wrist: difficulty in utilizing either primary or secondary MRI signs. J Comput Assist Tomogr 2001; 25(5):671.

107. Linkous MD, Pierce SD, Gilula LA. Scapholunate ligamentous communicating defects in symptomatic and asymptomatic wrists: characteristics 1. Radiology 2000;216(3):846–50.

108. Florkowski CM. Sensitivity, specificity, receiver-operating characteristic (ROC) curves and likelihood ratios: communicating the performance of diagnostic tests. Clin Biochem Rev 2008; 29(Suppl 1):S83–7.

109. Mayfield JK. Mechanism of carpal injuries. Clin Orthop Relat Res 1980;(149):45–54.

110. Mayfield JK. Patterns of Injury to Carpal Ligaments A Spectrum. Clin Orthop Relat Res 1984; 187:36.

111. Lee RK, Ng AW, Tong CS, et al. Intrinsic ligament and triangular fibrocartilage complex tears of the wrist: comparison of MDCT arthrography, conventional 3-T MRI, and MR arthrography. Skeletal Radiol 2013;42(9):1277–85.

112. Wright TW, Charco MD, Wheeler D. Incidence of ligament lesions and associated degenerative changes in the elderly wrist. J Hand Surg Am 1994;19(2):313–8.

113. Viegas SF, Patterson RM, Hokanson JA, et al. Wrist anatomy: incidence, distribution, and correlation of anatomic variations, tears, and arthrosis. J Hand Surg Am 1993;18(3):463–75.

114. Yin YM, Evanoff B, Gilula LA, et al. Evaluation of selective wrist arthrography of contralateral asymptomatic wrists for symmetric ligamentous

defects. AJR Am J Roentgenol 1996;166(5): 1067–73.

115. Brown JA, Janzen DL, Adler BD, et al. Arthrography of the contralateral, asymptomatic wrist in patients with unilateral wrist pain. Can Assoc Radiol J 1994;45(4):292–6.

116. Metz VM, Mann FA, Gilula LA. Lack of correlation between site of wrist pain and location of noncommunicating defects shown by three-compartment wrist arthrography. AJR Am J Roentgenol 1993; 160(6):1239–43.

117. Wilson AJ, Gilula LA, Mann FA. Unidirectional joint communications in wrist arthrography: an evaluation of 250 cases. AJR Am J Roentgenol 1991; 157(1):105–9.

118. Cantor RM, Stern PJ, Wyrick JD, et al. The relevance of ligament tears or perforations in the diagnosis of wrist pain: an arthrographic study. J Hand Surg Am 1994;19(6):945–53.

119. Kennedy SA, Allan CH. In brief: Mayfield et al. Classification: carpal dislocations and progressive perilunar instability. Clin Orthop Relat Res 2012; 470(4):1243–5.

120. Cerezal L, del Piñal F, Abascal F, et al. Imaging findings in ulnar-sided wrist impaction syndromes. Radiographics 2002;22(1):105–21.

121. Melone CP, Nathan R. Traumatic disruption of the triangular fibrocartilage complex. Pathoanatomy. Clin Orthop Relat Res 1992;275:65–73.

122. Wright TW, Dobyns JH, Linscheid RL, et al. Carpal instability non-dissociative. J Hand Surg Br 1994; 19(6):763–73.

123. Hash TW II. Magnetic resonance imaging of the knee. Sports Health 2013;5(1):78–107.

124. Lichtman DM, Wroten ES. Understanding mid-carpal instability. J Hand Surg Am 2006;31(3): 491–8.

125. Lichtman DM, Bruckner JD, Culp RW. Palmar mid-carpal instability: results of surgical reconstruction. J Hand Surg Am 1993;18(2):307–15.

126. Toms AP, Chojnowski A, Cahir JG. Midcarpal instability: a radiological perspective. Skeletal Radiol 2011;40(5):533–41.

127. Tay SC, Berger RA, Parker WL. Longitudinal split tears of the ulnotriquetral ligament. Hand Clin 2010;26(4):495–501.

128. Tay SC, Tomita K, Berger RA. The "ulnar fovea sign" for defining ulnar wrist pain: an analysis of sensitivity and specificity. J Hand Surg Am 2007;32(4):438–44.

129. Johnstone DJ, Thorogood S, Smith WH, et al. A comparison of magnetic resonance imaging and arthroscopy in the investigation of chronic wrist pain. J Hand Surg Br 1997;22(6):714–8.

130. Lee YH, Choi YR, Kim S, et al. Intrinsic ligament and triangular fibrocartilage complex (TFCC) tears of the wrist: comparison of isovolumetric 3D-THRIVE sequence MR arthrography and

conventional MR image at 3 T. Magn Reson Imaging 2013;31(2):221–6.

131. Spaans A, Minnen P, Prins H, et al. The value of 3.0-tesla MRI in diagnosing scapholunate ligament injury. J Wrist Surg 2013;02(01):69–72.

132. Schmitt R, Christopoulos G, Meier R. Direkte MR-Arthrographie des Handgelenks im Vergleich zur Arthroskopie: Eine prospektive Studie an 125 Patienten. Rofo 2003;175(7):911–9.

133. Hayden SR, Brown MD. Likelihood ratio: a powerful tool for incorporating the results of a diagnostic test into clinical decisionmaking. Ann Emerg Med 1999; 33(5):575–80.

134. Blazar PE, Chan PS, Kneeland JB, et al. The effect of observer experience on magnetic resonance imaging interpretation and localization of triangular fibrocartilage complex lesions. J Hand Surg Am 2001;26(4):742–8.

MR Imaging of the Triangular Fibrocartilage Complex

Michael E. Cody, MD[a], David T. Nakamura, MD[b],
Kirstin M. Small, MD[a], Hiroshi Yoshioka, MD, PhD[c],*

KEYWORDS

- Triangular fibrocartilage complex (TFCC) • 3D MR imaging • Wrist • Palmer classification

KEY POINTS

- The triangular fibrocartilage complex (TFCC) is an essential stabilizing structure of the wrist that is composed of numerous small components; an in-depth knowledge of its anatomy is essential to detect subtle pathologic conditions.
- Injuries of the TFCC may be acute or chronic and are often classified by the Palmer classification.
- Management of TFCC injury may include conservative, as well as surgical, treatments.
- Modern equipment and techniques such as high-resolution 2-dimensional (2D)/3-dimensional (3D) sequences, 3 T field strength, dedicated wrist coils, and direct arthrography may improve the ability to detect TFCC injury.

INTRODUCTION

Continued improvements in MR imaging allow greater detail than ever before. Thus, MR imaging is an invaluable tool in investigating injury of small anatomy, including the TFCC of the wrist. Accurate interpretation of wrist MR imaging requires knowledge of image acquisition techniques, thorough comprehension of the intricate anatomy, and understanding of common patterns of injury. Treatment of TFCC injury is in part predicated on the specific component of the TFCC that is injured as well as the acuity. Therefore, a precise description of TFCC injuries is valuable for treatment planning.

TECHNIQUE

Optimal imaging of the wrist requires maximizing spatial resolution, signal-to-noise ratio (SNR),
and contrast resolution. These variables are interconnected and influenced by changes in field of view (FOV), matrix size, slice thickness, bandwidth, echo time, repetition time, applied magnetic field strength, and pulse sequence selection.

High-spatial-resolution sequences are necessary to evaluate the fine structures that comprise the TFCC. In theory, increasing the matrix size for a given FOV or decreasing the FOV for a fixed matrix size can increase the spatial resolution. Such alterations result in loss of signal and subsequent degradation in image quality, which can be compensated for by adjusting other parameters (such as increasing applied field strength) or using specialized coils. Signal increase is approximately linear with increases in applied field, which can allow for increased resolution or decreases in scan time (with subsequent decreased risk of motion artifact). Specialized coils can also help

The authors have nothing to disclose.

[a] Department of Radiology, Brigham and Women's Hospital, 75 Francis Street, Boston, MA 02115, USA;
[b] Department of Radiology, UC Davis Medical Center, 4860 Y Street, Suite 3100, Sacramento, CA 95817, USA; [c] Department of Radiological Sciences, UC Irvine Medical Center, 101 The City Drive South, Route 140, Orange, CA 92868, USA

* Corresponding author.
E-mail address: hiroshi@uci.edu

Magn Reson Imaging Clin N Am 23 (2015) 393–403
http://dx.doi.org/10.1016/j.mric.2015.04.001
1064-9689/15/$ – see front matter © 2015 Elsevier Inc. All rights reserved.

augment signal. For example, it may be possible to use a specialized microscopy coil at 1.5 T and generate resolution similar to that of routine 3 T examinations.

The basic pulse sequence categories commonly used for imaging the wrist include proton density (PD)-weighted imaging, T2* gradient recalled echo sequences, and fluid-sensitive sequences with fat suppression. In general, sequences are acquired with conventional 2D technique, although 3D imaging techniques specific to the wrist have recently been described. The authors' routine wrist protocol includes coronal PD and PD fat-saturated, axial PD and PD fat-saturated, sagittal PD and PD fat-saturated, and coronal 3D PD and PD fat-saturated imaging (**Fig. 1**).

Three-dimensional MR imaging offers several advantages over conventional 2D sequences; 3D images with isotropic voxels can be reformatted into any cross-sectional plane from a single acquisition (**Fig. 2**). Structures can be cross-linked between planes without misregistration. Thinner slices reduce partial volume artifact because a lesion may be seen on multiple sequential slices. In addition, there is potential to decrease overall scan time because a single 3D coronal acquisition can be obtained followed by multiplanar reformats as opposed to obtaining separate orthogonal acquisitions as in conventional 2D imaging.

Designing a 3D imaging sequence for evaluation of the TFCC requires careful and specific optimization of multiple parameters, including scan time, echo train length (ETL), and inversion time (TI).[1] Increased slice thickness results in decreased scan time at the cost of increased image blur. Overall, decreasing ETL improves image blur. When scan time is held constant, decreasing slice thickness with a higher ETL results in less image blur. Decreased slice thickness and higher ETL may also result in incomplete fat suppression, which can be corrected by decreasing TIs.

Yamabe and colleagues[1] compared high-resolution conventional 2D fast spin echo and isotropic 3D PD and PD fat saturated MR images of the wrist at 3 T. Qualitative metrics evaluated included delineation of anatomic structures, amount of artifact, quality of fat suppression, image blur, and overall quality. Quantitative metrics were also evaluated, including relative signal intensity of each structure in the wrist and relative contrast between structures of the wrist. Their qualitative analysis found that for overall image quality, delineation of anatomic structures, and amount of artifact, there was no difference between 2D and 3D MR imaging. Although the study was limited to healthy volunteers and injury was not directly assessed, they did note that there were no significant differences in relative fluid to TFCC contrast between the 2 imaging sequences,

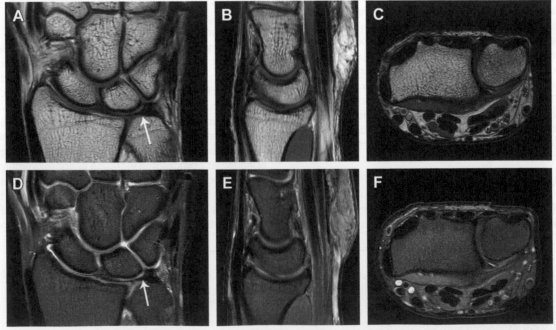

Fig. 1. Selected coronal (*A*), sagittal (*B*), and axial (*C*) 2D PD and coronal (*D*), sagittal (*E*), and axial (*F*) 2D PD fat-saturated images of the wrist using routine sequences. Note the central disk of the TFCC (*arrows*), which is easiest to evaluate in the coronal plane.

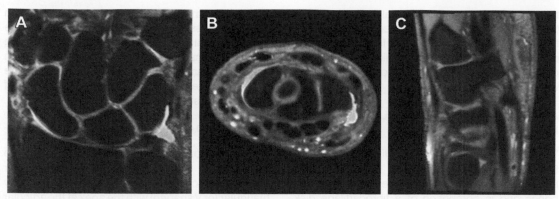

Fig. 2. Coronal 3D isotropic PD fat-saturated sequence (*A*). Isotropic voxels allow for reformations in any plane, including standard axial (*B*) and sagittal (*C*) reformats.

inferring that 3D and 2D imaging sequences may have similar detection rates for TFCC pathology.

Direct MR arthrography (MRA), involving intra-articular injection of dilute gadolinium contrast, is an accurate and established method for evaluating TFCC pathology.[2,3] Arthrography results in distention of the joint capsule and supporting ligaments, allowing for direct visualization. In addition, there is improved contrast resolution between the high-signal gadolinium contrast and low-signal structures of the TFCC. MRA is also useful for verifying full-thickness TFCC tears, which are demonstrated by contrast extravasation into the distal radioulnar joint (DRUJ) in single-compartment radiocarpal arthrography. In addition, tear of the capsule or ulnar collateral ligament complex can be similarly visualized as contrast extravasation (**Fig. 3**). Downsides of MRA compared with traditional MR imaging include additional cost and time, discomfort for the patient, and small risk of infection, bleeding, or contrast reaction.

Lee and colleagues[4] recently evaluated a fast T1-weighted 3D sequence called 3D T1 high-resolution isotropic volume examination (3D-THRIVE) for the detection of central and peripheral TFCC tears. Patients in the study underwent routine 2D PD and T2-weighted MR imaging followed by arthrography and 3D-THRIVE MRA. The results of the imaging studies were compared to arthroscopy as the gold standard. Sensitivity for 3D MRA was 94.6% for central TFCC tears and 93.3% for peripheral tears compared with 2D MR imaging sensitivities of 70.3% for central TFCC tears and 60% for peripheral TFCC tears. In addition to improved sensitivity, total acquisition time for 3D MRA was shorter, averaging only 3 minutes, 40 seconds for coronal sequences.

Indirect arthrography is a technique in which a standard dose of 0.1 mmol/kg of gadolinium-based contrast is injected intravenously in lieu of direct intra-articular puncture, allowing contrast

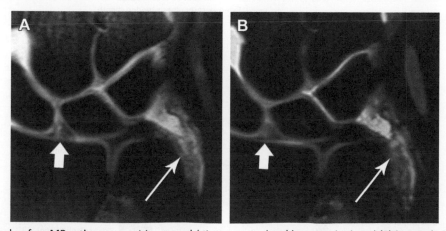

Fig. 3. Sample of an MR arthrogram with coronal (*A*) FS T1-wieghted imaging (WI) and (*B*) isotropic 3D FS PD-WI sequences. Note massive contrast leak through prestyloid recess signifying tear of the ulnar collateral ligament complex of the TFCC (*thin arrows*). In addition, there is also a tear of the scapholunate ligament, allowing contrast into the midcarpal row (*thick arrows*).

to accumulate within the synovial fluid after a brief (5–10 minute) delay. Haims and colleagues[5] investigated the use of indirect MRA for the evaluation of TFCC central disk tears, finding no significant difference in sensitivity or specificity compared with unenhanced MR imaging.

ANATOMY OF THE TRIANGULAR FIBROCARTILAGE COMPLEX

The TFCC is an essential stabilizing structure of the DRUJ and ulnar carpus. The TFCC is centered between the distal ulna and the proximal carpal bones and is composed of a fibrocartilage disk and multiple surrounding ligaments.[6] There is some controversy about the exact components of the TFCC, but for the purposes of this article, the complex is composed of TFC disproper, triangular ligament, ulnar collateral ligament, ulnotriquetral ligament, ulnolunate ligament, and the meniscus homologue (**Fig. 4**).

The TFC proper is composed of the dorsal and volar radioulnar ligaments and the fibrocartilage central disk.[7] The components of the TFC proper attach to the distal radius. Typically, the fibrocartilage central disk is considered the focal point of the TFCC and is regarded as an asymmetric four-sided structure with concave facets (tetracuspid). The TFCC may be further divided into its volar and dorsal as well as radial and ulnar components.

RADIAL ATTACHMENT

There is a broad attachment of the TFCC to the radius, with the dorsal and volar radioulnar ligaments inserting on the radius at the periphery of the central fibrocartilage disk at the level of the

sigmoid notch. The radioulnar ligaments attach at bony entheses at the volar and dorsal aspects of the distal radius, while the central fibrocartilage disk transitions into the hyaline cartilage between these two ligaments. Coronal images demonstrate curvilinear intermediate signal at this transition of the central disk and the hyaline cartilage.

ULNAR ATTACHMENT

The connection between the central fibrocartilage disk and the ulna occurs through the triangular ligament, which, as its name suggests, is roughly triangular (or V shaped) with the apex at the articular disk and its base occurring at the distal ulna. The triangular ligament has a striated appearance on MR imaging because of its underlying collagen fiber composition. Near its attachment on the ulna, the triangular ligament typically bifurcates into two laminae, which attach at the distal tip of the ulnar styloid and more proximally at the ulnar fovea. These two bands of the triangular ligament are often separated by relatively increased signal tissue called the ligamentum subcruentum. The more proximal fibers of the distal lamina of the triangular ligament become intimately involved with the ulnar joint capsule. In addition, the ulnotriquetral and ulnolunate ligaments lie at the volar aspect of the TFCC, while the extensor carpi ulnaris subsheath is at the dorsal ulnar aspect of the complex.

VASCULARITY OF THE TRIANGULAR FIBROCARTILAGE COMPLEX

Most of the blood supply to the TFCC is via the ulnar artery, directly and indirectly. Like the menisci of the knee, the central portion of the

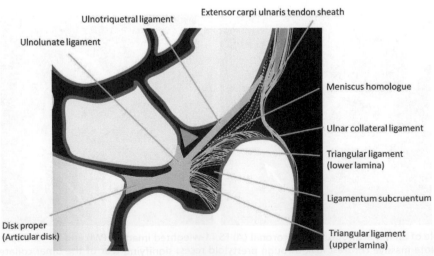

Fig. 4. Schematic illustrating the components of the TFCC. (*From* Yoshioka H, Burns JE. Magnetic resonance imaging of triangular fibrocartilage. J Magn Reson Imaging 2012;35(4):770; with permission.)

TFCC and its more radial attachments are relatively avascular, whereas the periphery of the disk is more vascular.[8] Similar to the knee meniscus, injury to the relatively avascular portions has less potential for healing and repair. At the most ulnar aspect of the TFCC near the styloid process, the ulnar artery proper supplies most of the blood through penetrating end vessels. More radially, the TFCC receives blood through dorsal and volar branches of the anterior interosseous artery, an early branch vessel of the ulnar artery distal to the elbow.

TRIANGULAR FIBROCARTILAGE COMPLEX INJURY
MR Imaging of Triangular Fibrocartilage Complex Injury

Multiple studies have shown that MR imaging is useful in the evaluation of TFCC injuries.[9–13] Magee[10] evaluated the sensitivity and specificity of 3 T MR imaging and MRA for the evaluation of TFCC tears. He found that the MR imaging sensitivity for the detection of TFCC tears was 86% and the specificity was 100% with no false-positive results. The sensitivity for detection of TFCC tears on MRA was 100%. A few false-positive results were found on MRA in which contrast passed between the radiocarpal and DRUJ spaces without TFCC tear identified. Arthroscopy performed on these cases did not demonstrate any tears, suggesting underlying microperforations.

The magnetic field strength may play a role in MR imaging accuracy for the detection of TFCC lesions. Anderson and colleagues[9] compared the diagnostic performance of preoperative MR imaging at 1.5 T and 3 T with that of wrist arthroscopy, finding a trend toward improved sensitivity, specificity, and accuracy at 3 T. Imaging at 3 T offers higher SNR, which in theory should allow for improved imaging quality at a given spatial resolution.

Despite the use of MR imaging as a noninvasive test for the detection of TFCC pathology, there are certain lesions that are difficult to visualize on MR imaging. In particular, peripheral tears at the ulnar attachment of the TFCC remain difficult to accurately diagnose on MR imaging. Haims and colleagues[14] found that if ligamentous disruption is used as the evidence for ulnar attachment tear, the sensitivity for the detection of peripheral tears of the TFCC was 17%, with a specificity of 79% and an accuracy of 64%. When high signal intensity was used as the marker for peripheral tear, they found that the sensitivity improved to 42%, whereas the specificity and accuracy dropped to 63% and 55%, respectively.

Abnormalities of the TFCC on MR imaging can be seen in asymptomatic wrists. A recent study by Iordache and colleagues[15] found that the prevalence of TFCC lesions in asymptomatic volunteers was 37.9%. Complete tears of the TFCC were seen in 22.3% wrists with a trend toward increased prevalence of abnormalities with increased age. This trend is in agreement with early cadaveric studies that demonstrated that degeneration and subsequent perforations increased with age, reaching up to 53% of wrists in the seventh decade.[16]

Mechanism of Injury and Symptoms

Patients with TFCC pathology may present with diffuse wrist or ulnar-sided pain, which may be accompanied by mechanical symptoms such as clicking or snapping sensations with rotation. The most common mechanism of traumatic injury to the TFCC is axial load to an extended wrist with forearm pronation, which can occur with a fall onto an outstretched hand. Distraction forces applied to the volar wrist, common in racket sports, can also predispose to TFCC injury. The structures of the TFCC, including the dorsal and palmar radioulnar ligaments, are crucial stabilizers to the DRUJ, and injury to these structures can result in DRUJ instability. Anatomic factors such as positive ulnar variance can predispose patients to both acute injuries and chronic degenerative processes.

Classification

The Palmer classification divides TFCC tears as traumatic (Class 1) and degenerative (Class 2) (**Table 1**).[17] This system is frequently used by hand surgeons and can help direct clinical management.[11] Although knowledge of this system is useful, it is important to recognize that the classification is not exhaustive and does not encompass all components of the TFCC. In addition, not all TFCC injuries neatly fit into this classification system.

Traumatic Triangular Fibrocartilage Complex Tears

Palmer Class 1 tears are subclassified according to the location of injury. Class 1A tears involve a tear or perforation of the central fibrocartilage disk and are the most common traumatic subtype of TFCC tear (**Fig. 5**).[18] Despite being classified as central perforations, the tear often occurs at the radial half of the disk (but not immediately abutting the hyaline cartilage overlying the sigmoid notch at the radial attachment, a Class 1D lesion). Tears may also have complex configuration, analogous

Table 1	
Palmer classification of TFCC abnormalities	
Class 1: Traumatic	**Class 2: Degenerative**
A. Central perforation	A. TFCC wear
B. Ulnar avulsion distal ulnar fracture	B. TFCC wear + lunate and/or ulnar chondromalacia
C. Distal avulsion	C. TFCC perforation + lunate and/or ulnar chondromalacia
D. Radial avulsion sigmoid notch fracture	D. TFCC perforation + lunate and/or ulnar chondromalacia + lunotriquetral ligament perforation
	E. TFCC perforation + lunate and/or ulnar chondromalacia + lunotriquetral ligament perforation + ulnocarpal arthritis

From Palmer AK. Triangular fibrocartilage complex lesions: a classification. J Hand Surg 1989;14(4):596, with permission.

to complex tears of the knee meniscus (**Fig. 6**). Class 1B lesions are peripheral tears of the TFCC near or at its insertion on the distal ulna. These tears may involve purely ligamentous avulsions from the ulnar attachments of the TFCC (**Fig. 7**) or fracture through the base of the ulnar styloid process and are often accompanied by DRUJ instability. Tears of the ulnar attachment (triangular ligament) are particularly difficult to accurately diagnose because striated fascicles associated with the ligamentum subcruentum may mask or mimic tears. Class 1C lesions, referred to as distal avulsions, involve tears of the volar ligaments, specifically the ulnolunate or ulnotriquetral ligaments (**Fig. 8**). These ligaments are robust and therefore relatively resistant to this type of injury making Class 1C lesions uncommon. These injuries can result in ulnar carpal instability with palmar migration of the ulnar carpus. Finally, Class 1D lesions involve avulsion of the TFCC from its radial attachment at the sigmoid notch of the radius. These injuries may involve avulsion fracture of the sigmoid notch. As opposed to central (Class 1A) lesions in which fluid signal is confined to the TFCC disk proper, in radial avulsions, abnormal fluid signal extends between the radial attachment of the TFCC and the hyaline cartilage of the distal radius.

Although the Palmer classification is useful in characterizing TFCC injuries, it must be reemphasized that many TFCC injuries fall outside of this classification system.[19] For instance, injury of the extensor carpi ulnaris tendon sheath, the ulnar collateral ligament complex (as seen in **Fig. 3**), and volar and dorsal radioulnar ligaments are not accounted for by this system. Because injury to the TFCC often includes several of its constituent elements, care should be taken to avoid satisfaction of search when evaluating this complex structure. It is also advisable to describe each lesion independent of the Palmer classification before trying to categorize the injury.

Degenerative Triangular Fibrocartilage Complex Injury

Degenerative, or Class 2, lesions are caused by chronic loading of the ulnar wrist, such as that seen in ulnar impaction syndrome, and are classified according to the extent of degeneration and surrounding secondary changes. Class 2A lesions involve wear or thinning of the central disk without perforation. Class 2B lesions similarly involve thinning of the disk and also include lunate and/or ulnar head chondromalacia. Class 2C lesions involve further progression with perforation of the TFCC and include lunate and/or ulnar head chondromalacia (**Fig. 9**). Perforations in the setting of degeneration differ from traumatic tears in that perforations tend to be more ovoid in configuration and typically located more toward the ulnar aspect of the fibrocartilage disk. Class 2D lesions involve TFCC perforation with lunate and/or ulnar chondromalacia and lunotriquetral ligament disruption. Finally, Class 2E lesions involve ulnocarpal and occasionally DRUJ degenerative arthritis in addition to the abnormalities encompassed by Class 2D. By this stage of degeneration, the fibrocartilage disk is often entirely absent or extensively macerated.

Degeneration

Degeneration of the TFCC progresses with age. Pathologic changes include mucoid degeneration, fibrillation, and abnormal thinning.[16] On MR imaging, these pathologic changes are demonstrated as increased, intermediate curvilinear, or globular signal intensity within the TFCC without surface communication (**Fig. 10**).

Pitfalls

Rotation of the wrist can result in subtle morphologic variation of the TFCC. For example, on pronation, there can be apparent thinning of the central disk in the coronal plane.[20] In the absence of substantial signal alteration, this finding should not be interpreted as pathologic.

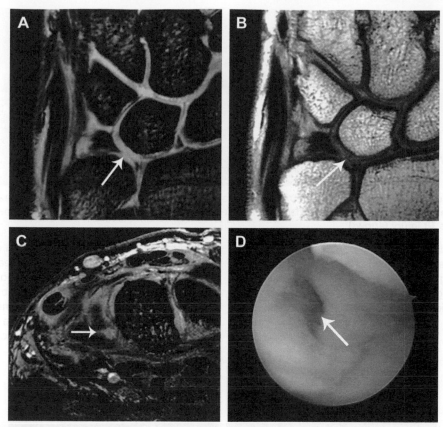

Fig. 5. TFCC central perforation (Palmer Class 1A lesion). Coronal gradient recalled echo (GRE) image (*A*) and PD-weighted image (*B*) demonstrate the defect of the central disk, which normally shows bow-tie-like low signal intensity. Axial GRE image (*C*) also shows central disk injury as a geographic high-signal-intensity area consistent with arthroscopic (*D*) findings (*arrows*). (*From* Tanaka T, Ogino S, Yoshioka H. Ligamentous injuries of the wrist. Semin Musculoskelet Radiol 2008;12(4):362; with permission.)

As discussed previously, the ligamentum subcruentum is a vascular tissue that separates the 2 lamina of the triangular ligament at the distal ulnar attachment. This tissue often demonstrates intermediate or increased PD signal. In contrast to perforation or a tear of the triangular ligament, in which the signal extends into or through the collagen fibrils, the ligamentum subcruentum is a

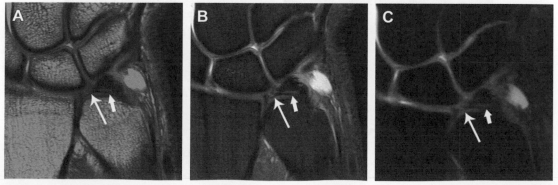

Fig. 6. Two-dimensional coronal PD (*A*), 2D coronal PD fat-saturated (*B*), and 3D isotropic PD fat-saturated (*C*) images demonstrate complex tear involving the TFCC articular disk with vertical component (*thin arrows*) and horizontal component extending to the periphery (*thick arrows*).

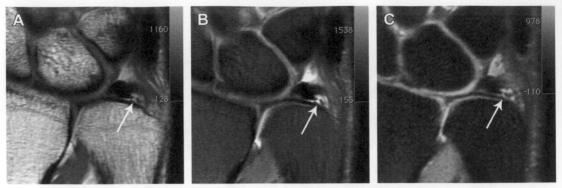

Fig. 7. Two-dimensional coronal PD (*A*), 2D coronal PD fat-saturated (*B*), and 3D isotropic PD fat-saturated (*C*) images demonstrate a partial tear of the triangular ligament near the ulnar foveal attachment/proximal lamina, a Palmer Class 1B injury (*arrows*).

normal finding and should be fully surrounded by the laminae and distal ulna on coronal images. In challenging cases, the authors have found that reformatting their coronal 3D isotropic sequence into an oblique coronal plane is helpful in differentiating tear from normal attachments (**Fig. 11**).

Intermediate signal within the central disk of the TFCC does not necessarily indicate tear. As with the menisci of the knee, intermediate nonsurfacing signal within the substance of the fibrocartilage disk is commonly seen and represents intrinsic degeneration rather than tear. Extensive degeneration and/or signal alteration from chondrocalcinosis,

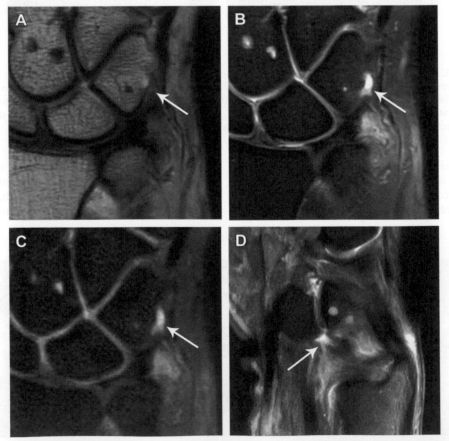

Fig. 8. Two-dimensional coronal PD (*A*), 2D coronal PD fat-saturated (*B*), coronal 3D volume isotropic turbo spin echo acquisition (*C*), and sagittal PD fat-saturated (*D*) images demonstrate tear of the ulnotriquetral ligament (*arrows*). This lesion would be classified as Palmer Class 1C.

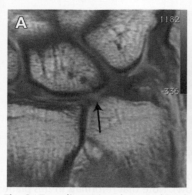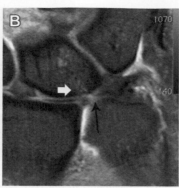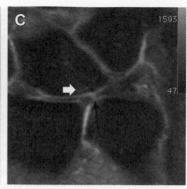

Fig. 9. Two-dimensional coronal PD (*A*), 2D coronal PD fat-saturated (*B*), and 3D isotropic PD fat-saturated (*C*) images demonstrate diffuse intermediate signal with attenuation of the central disk and focal full-thickness defect (*black thin arrows*) consistent with degenerative tear with adjacent cartilage thinning and subchondral edema of the lunate (*white thick arrows*). This constellation of findings is compatible with a Palmer Class 2C abnormality.

such as with calcium pyrophosphate dihydrate (CPPD) deposition, may mimic Palmer Class 2 lesions, and correlation with radiographs or computed tomographic images is prudent in this setting before diagnosing a tear of the TFCC.

The hyaline cartilage of the sigmoid notch at the distal radius has intermediate signal intensity and is an attachment site for the central portion of the fibrocartilage disk. The intrinsic curvilinear intermediate signal of the hyaline cartilage-fibrocartilage interface should not be mistaken for a tear or injury of the radial attachment of the TFCC. The normal interface can be distinguished from a Palmer Class 2D lesion because it does not demonstrate gadolinium (arthrography) or fluid signal and it is smoothly marginated.

Management of Triangular Fibrocartilage Complex Injury

Initial treatment of both acute and chronic TFCC injuries is generally nonoperative using a combination of rest, immobilization, physical rehabilitation/therapy, and/or corticosteroid injection. Some clinicians have argued that long cast immobilization in neutral position may be appropriate. However, in patients who remain symptomatic after these conservative measures, surgery may be necessary.

There are numerous surgical approaches to TFCC injury, but they can generally be divided into open and arthroscopic procedures with debridement and/or repair. Repair of the TFCC usually includes some level of debridement at the margin of the injury, which is thought to induce bleeding, in turn, stimulating healing. TFCC repair is typically reserved for patients with acute TFCC injury or athletes who require definitive treatment to return to play. In addition, central disk injury, whether acute or chronic, is thought to have overall worse outcomes with repair rather than debridement because of the relatively diminished blood supply to this area. The corollary is that peripheral TFCC injuries may demonstrate improved healing because of the relatively

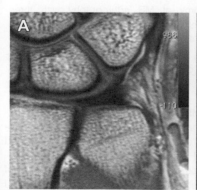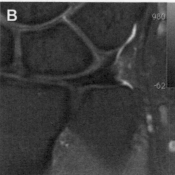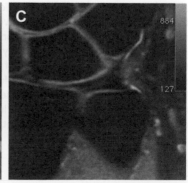

Fig. 10. Two-dimensional coronal PD (*A*), 2D coronal PD fat-saturated (*B*), and 3D isotropic PD fat-saturated (*C*) images demonstrate intermediate nonsurfacing signals within the disk proper compatible with degeneration without tear.

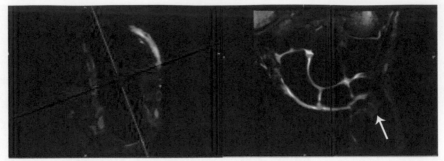

Fig. 11. Axial (*left*) and oblique coronal (*right*) multiplanar reconstruction from coronal 3D isotropic PD fat-saturated images demonstrating intact ulnar attachments of the TFCC (*arrow*). Note that reformats in this plane can aid in the visualization of the ulnar attachments of the TFCC, which is a particularly challenging area to evaluate.

increased vascularity. Proponents of arthroscopic technique suggest that because of the limited nature of the incisions required for portals, there is improved visualization of the injury, decreased injury to surrounding tissues, and improved wrist motion.[21] Some argue that only open surgery provides definitive reattachment of the TFCC foveal connections. However, there is no reported significant difference in outcomes between open and arthroscopic techniques with regard to range of motion, grip strength, pain, or reoperation rate for DRUJ instability.[22] Positive ulnar variance has been associated with increased failure of arthroscopic debridement procedures. Ulnar variance may be addressed at the time of TFCC repair/debridement if needed, such as with ulnocarpal unloading procedures.

SUMMARY

MR imaging is useful in the evaluation of the TFCC because of excellent soft tissue contrast and improvements in resolution allowing for thorough evaluation of the small structures that constitute the TFCC. MR imaging provides valuable information to the hand surgeon by delineating location and extent of tears and allowing for preoperative treatment planning. While conventional pulse sequences with 2D acquisition comprise the bulk of imaging techniques in use today, new developments allow for acquisition of 3D isotropic sequences in clinically acceptable time frames. While still under investigation, these techniques may prove useful in detection of injuries that are difficult to evaluate on routine sequences.

REFERENCES

1. Yamabe E, Anavim A, Sakai T, et al. Comparison between high-resolution isotropic three-dimensional and high-resolution conventional two-dimensional FSE MR images of the wrist at 3 Tesla: a pilot study. J Magn Reson Imaging 2014;40(3):603–8.
2. Lee RK, Ng AW, Tong CS, et al. Intrinsic ligament and triangular fibrocartilage complex tears of the wrist: comparison of MDCT arthrography, conventional 3-T MRI, and MR arthrography. Skeletal Radiol 2013;42(9):1277–85.
3. Zanetti M, Bram J, Hodler J. Triangular fibrocartilage and intercarpal ligaments of the wrist: does MR arthrography improve standard MRI? J Magn Reson Imaging 1997;7(3):590–4.
4. Lee YH, Choi YR, Kim S, et al. Intrinsic ligament and triangular fibrocartilage complex (TFCC) tears of the wrist: comparison of isovolumetric 3D-THRIVE sequence MR arthrography and conventional MR image at 3 T. Magn Reson Imag 2013; 31(2):221–6.
5. Haims AH, Schweitzer ME, Morrison WB, et al. Internal derangement of the wrist: indirect MR arthrography versus unenhanced MR imaging. Radiology 2003;227(3):701–7.
6. Vezeridis PS, Yoshioka H, Han R, et al. Ulnar-sided wrist pain. Part I: anatomy and physical examination. Skeletal Radiol 2010;39(8):733–45.
7. Brown RR, Fliszar E, Cotten A, et al. Extrinsic and intrinsic ligaments of the wrist: normal and pathologic anatomy at MR arthrography with three-compartment enhancement. Radiographics 1998; 18(3):667–74.
8. Bednar MS, Arnoczky SP, Weiland AJ. The microvasculature of the triangular fibrocartilage complex: its clinical significance. J Hand Surg 1991;16(6):1101–5.
9. Anderson ML, Skinner JA, Felmlee JP, et al. Diagnostic comparison of 1.5 Tesla and 3.0 Tesla preoperative MRI of the wrist in patients with ulnar-sided wrist pain. J Hand Surg 2008;33(7):1153–9.
10. Magee T. Comparison of 3-T MRI and arthroscopy of intrinsic wrist ligament and TFCC tears. AJR Am J Roentgenol 2009;192(1):80–5.
11. Oneson SR, Scales LM, Timins ME, et al. MR imaging interpretation of the Palmer classification of

triangular fibrocartilage complex lesions. Radiographics 1996;16(1):97–106.

12. Potter HG, Asnis-Ernberg L, Weiland AJ, et al. The utility of high-resolution magnetic resonance imaging in the evaluation of the triangular fibrocartilage complex of the wrist. J Bone Joint Surg Am 1997; 79(11):1675–84.

13. Tanaka T, Yoshioka H, Ueno T, et al. Comparison between high-resolution MRI with a microscopy coil and arthroscopy in triangular fibrocartilage complex injury. J Hand Surg 2006;31(8):1308–14.

14. Haims AH, Schweitzer ME, Morrison WB, et al. Limitations of MR imaging in the diagnosis of peripheral tears of the triangular fibrocartilage of the wrist. AJR Am J Roentgenol 2002;178(2):419–22.

15. Iordache SD, Rowan R, Garvin GJ, et al. Prevalence of triangular fibrocartilage complex abnormalities on MRI scans of asymptomatic wrists. J Hand Surg 2012;37(1):98–103.

16. Mikic ZD. Age changes in the triangular fibrocartilage of the wrist joint. J Anat 1978;126(Pt 2):367–84.

17. Palmer AK. Triangular fibrocartilage complex lesions: a classification. J Hand Surg 1989;14(4):594–606.

18. Sachar K. Ulnar-sided wrist pain: evaluation and treatment of triangular fibrocartilage complex tears, ulnocarpal impaction syndrome, and lunotriquetral ligament tears. J Hand Surg 2008;33(9):1669–79.

19. Daunt N. Magnetic resonance imaging of the wrist: anatomy and pathology of interosseous ligaments and the triangular fibrocartilage complex. Curr Probl Diagn Radiol 2002;31(4):158–76.

20. Burns JE, Tanaka T, Ueno T, et al. Pitfalls that may mimic injuries of the triangular fibrocartilage and proximal intrinsic wrist ligaments at MR imaging. Radiographics 2011;31(1):63–78.

21. Bednar JM, Osterman AL. The role of arthroscopy in the treatment of traumatic triangular fibrocartilage injuries. Hand Clin 1994;10(4):605–14.

22. Anderson ML, Larson AN, Moran SL, et al. Clinical comparison of arthroscopic versus open repair of triangular fibrocartilage complex tears. J Hand Surg 2008;33(5):675–82.

MR Imaging of Carpal Fractures

Naveen S. Murthy, MD*, Michael D. Ringler, MD

KEYWORDS

- MRI • Fractures • Osteonecrosis • Scaphoid • Carpal bones • Triquetrum • Hamate

KEY POINTS

- The early diagnosis of carpal fractures is critical for appropriate, timely management to minimize complications related to delayed diagnosis such as fracture progression, nonunion, osteonecrosis, and secondary degenerative arthritis.
- In the setting of an acute wrist injury, the American College of Radiology (ACR) recommends radiography as the initial imaging modality, with a specialized carpal tunnel view in suspected hook of the hamate fractures.
- On obtaining negative results on initial radiographs, early magnetic resonance (MR) imaging can exclude carpal fracture.
- When a carpal fracture is excluded, MR imaging can also provide alternative diagnoses, such as other unsuspected fractures involving the distal radius/ulna or hand, osseous contusions, and soft-tissue injuries.
- MR imaging is the imaging modality of choice to assess the viability of the proximal fragment in scaphoid nonunion. Unfortunately, the imaging protocol is not universally agreed upon.

INTRODUCTION

The early diagnosis of carpal fractures is important for appropriate, timely management of these injuries. Potential complications related to delayed or missed diagnosis include fracture progression, nonunion, osteonecrosis, and secondary degenerative arthritis.[1] There may also be a substantial cost associated with lost work productivity related to a delayed diagnosis.[1]

The ACR has developed Appropriateness Criteria (AC)[2] to help identify the most appropriate imaging studies that should be performed for a particular suspected condition. The AC have been developed for nearly every major organ system by a panel of experts on the subject, using all available literature to date. Based on this body of evidence, the expert panel assigned a number for the various imaging modalities indicating the appropriateness of the test in various stages of the workup of the suspected condition. A 1 to 9 rating scale is used: 1, 2, and 3 are usually not appropriate; 4, 5, and 6 may be appropriate; 7, 8, and 9 are usually appropriate.[2] When ionizing radiation is used, the AC also provide the relative radiation levels for the imaging modalities. Fortunately, ionizing radiation imparted to the adult wrist by either radiography or computed tomography (CT) is small, on the order of 0.1 mSv.[2] In comparison, the average yearly background radiation in the United States is approximately 30 times this amount.[3] In the setting of an acute wrist injury, the ACR recommends radiography as the initial modality in the workup (AC rating 9).[2] Standard 2 views are not sufficient, with up to 4 views preferred and additional views obtained as

The authors have nothing to disclose.
Division of Musculoskeletal Radiology, Department of Radiology, Mayo Clinic, 200 First Street Southwest, Rochester, MN 55905, USA
* Corresponding author.
E-mail address: murthy.naveen@mayo.edu

Magn Reson Imaging Clin N Am 23 (2015) 405–416
http://dx.doi.org/10.1016/j.mric.2015.04.006
1064-9689/15/$ – see front matter © 2015 Elsevier Inc. All rights reserved.

necessary depending on the suspected fracture.[2] Unfortunately, in cases in which the carpal fracture is radiographically occult, further evaluation is required. MR imaging can provide early diagnosis of carpal fractures with the added benefit of not imparting ionizing radiation. In addition, MR imaging can provide alternative diagnoses when a carpal fracture is not identified, such as other noncarpal fractures, osseous contusions, and soft-tissue injuries, including intrinsic and extrinsic ligamentous pathology (MR Imaging of Wrist Ligaments by Ringler and colleagues). For the latter diagnoses, high spatial resolution and signal to noise ratio is required, facilitated by a field strength of 1.5 T or higher. In a recent publication, 136 consecutive patients with suspected, radiographically occult, scaphoid fractures were studied.[1] Within 7 days of initial presentation with negative results on radiographs, 1.5-T MRI was performed. A total of 16 (11.7%) patients had scaphoid fractures, whereas 14 (10.3%) had fractures of other carpal bones or the distal radius, 55 (40.4%) had osseous contusions, and 50 (43.4%) had soft-tissue injuries.[1]

IMAGING

At the authors' institution, MR imaging of the wrist is commonly performed at 3 T (GE 750w, GE Healthcare, Waukesha, WI), using a birdcage coil developed in house. The MR imaging protocols used are listed in **Table 1**. The full MR imaging protocol for evaluation of the wrist in suspected carpal injuries includes 3 planes (axial, sagittal, and coronal) of T1-weighted and T2-weighted with fat saturation sequences. The limited protocol, used specifically for fractures or osseous contusion of the carpal bones, generally consists of coronal and sagittal T2-weighted with fat saturation sequences of the wrist to assess for bone marrow edema signal related to injury. A T1-weighted plane, sagittal or coronal, is added to assist in assessing for a linear low-signal-intensity abnormality, connoting a fracture line. One major advantage for developing a limited imaging protocol is monetary. At the authors' institution, the cost of a limited protocol is approximately 1 to 1.5 times that of a noncontrast extremity CT, whereas a full protocol examination is approximately 2 times the cost of a noncontrast extremity CT.

Regardless of protocol, the presence or absence of bone marrow edema signal is the key to an acute or subacute osseous injury. If there is no intramedullary T2-hyperintensity, an acute fracture and osseous contusion can be confidently excluded (**Fig. 1A**). When a discrete linear low-signal-intensity abnormality is identified, with surrounding bone marrow edema signal, a fracture can be confidently diagnosed (see **Fig. 1B**). If there is a band of bone marrow edema signal, without a discrete linear low-signal-intensity abnormality, this is consistent with microtrabecular injury or osseous contusion (see **Fig. 1C**). The distinction between a nondisplaced fracture and a contusion may have consequences regarding treatment, including potential surgical intervention, length of immobilization, and follow-up.[4,5] Osseous contusions do not require surgical intervention, but

Parameter	Axial T1 FSE	Axial T2FS FSE	Sagittal T1 FSE	Sagittal T2FS FSE	Coronal T1 FSE	Coronal T2FS FSE
Full protocol	X	X	X	X	X	X
Limited protocol	—	—	Optional	X	Optional	X
TR (ms)	700–900	3000–6000	700–900	3000–6000	700–900	3000–6000
TE (ms)	Min.	45	Min.	45	Min.	45
Echo train length	2	10	3	12	3	10
Bandwidth (kHz)	32	32	32	32	32	32
Matrix	384/256	384/256	384/256	384/256	384/256	384/256
FOV (cm)	10	10	10	10	10	10
NEX	2	2	2	2	2	2
Section thickness (mm)	3	3	2	2	2	2
Skip (mm)	0	0	0	0	0	0

Table 1
Three-tesla MR imaging protocols of the wrist

Abbreviations: FOV, field of view; FS, fat saturated; FSE, fast spin echo; Min., minimum; NEX, number of excitations; TE, echo time; TR, repetition time.

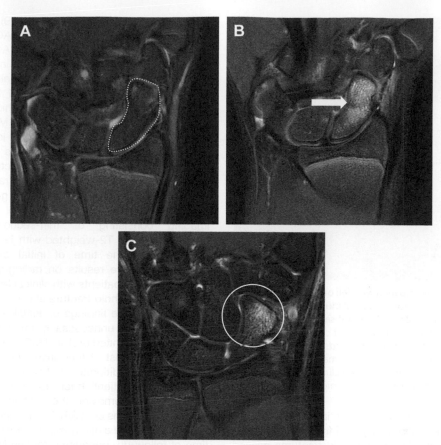

Fig. 1. Coronal T2-weighted fat-saturated MR images through the scaphoid. (*A*) There is no bone marrow edema within the scaphoid (*dotted white outline*); therefore, fracture and contusion are excluded. (*B*) There is a discrete linear low signal intensity through the waist of the scaphoid (*arrow*) with surrounding bone marrow edema, consistent with a fracture. (*C*) There is feathery bone marrow edema within the distal pole of the scaphoid (*circle*) without a discrete linear low signal intensity, compatible with an osseous contusion.

they may require immobilization and follow-up. One study found that, of 50 patients with osseous contusions of the scaphoid diagnosed with MR imaging, 2% progressed to a fracture despite plaster immobilization for 8 weeks.[4] However, another study found no progression of osseous contusion of the scaphoid to fracture with 6 weeks of immobilization.[5]

MR imaging can also help assess fracture acuity in cases in which the history is difficult to ascertain. Fractures with prominent surrounding bone marrow edema signal typically represent acute injuries. Fractures with little or no surrounding bone marrow edema are usually chronic injuries (**Fig. 2**). Although there are no studies to date specifically on bone marrow edema and the acuity of the injury in the appendicular skeleton, there is 1 study pertaining to the axial skeleton.[6] This group of investigators found that acute vertebral body compression fractures reliably generate bone marrow edema, whereas acute fractures that occur

in distraction do not reliably generate bone marrow edema.[6] These mechanisms should be considered in assessing for carpal fractures on MR imaging.

SCAPHOID FRACTURES

Scaphoid fractures account for 58% to 89% of all carpal fractures[7–10] and can be complicated by nonunion in 10% to 12% of cases.[11,12] The most common mechanism of injury is a fall onto an outstretched hand, resulting in wrist dorsiflexion, imparting palmar tensile and dorsal compressive forces on the scaphoid.[10]

Diagnosis

The most appropriate imaging study for the initial evaluation of suspected acute scaphoid fracture is radiography, according to the ACR AC (**Fig. 3**).[2] Radiographs should include at least 4 views: posteroanterior (PA), lateral, semipronated oblique, and PA with ulnar deviation.[2] In a

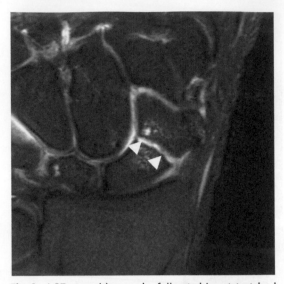

Fig. 2. A 37-year-old man who fell onto his outstretched right hand in the shower several months before presentation. Coronal T2-weighted fat-saturated MR image through the scaphoid shows a well-corticated un-united scaphoid waist fracture (*arrowheads*) without a substantial amount of surrounding bone marrow edema. These findings in conjunction with the clinical time frame are compatible with a scaphoid nonunion.

large meta-analysis, 84% of initial radiographs correctly identified a scaphoid fracture or no fracture.[13] About 16% of scaphoid fractures missed on the initial radiographs were diagnosed with follow-up radiography.[13] Therefore, if the initial radiographs are negative for a suspected acute scaphoid fracture, the ACR AC recommends noncontrast MR imaging (AC rating 9), cast and repeat radiographs in 10 to 14 days (AC rating 8), or noncontrast CT without contrast (AC rating 7) (see **Fig. 3**). Noncontrast MR imaging in the evaluation of suspected, radiographically occult, scaphoid fracture has a sensitivity of 100%,[13–15] specificity of 95% to 100%,[13–15] and high interobserver reliability ($\kappa = 0.8$–0.96).[13,14,16] MR imaging may also be more cost-effective, at least in the United States. Dorsay and colleagues[17] were the first group to publish the cost-effectiveness of MR imaging in the early evaluation of radiographically occult scaphoid fractures. This group of investigators used a limited protocol 1.5-T MR imaging consisting of thin-section coronal T1-weighted and T2-weighted with fat saturation sequences at the time of initial presentation following negative results on radiographs. They found that 3 of 4 patients with clinical findings suggestive of a scaphoid fracture at clinical examination, and negative findings on initial radiographs, were potentially unnecessarily immobilized and monitored.[17] A limited protocol MR imaging examination of the wrist at their institution cost $770, whereas the traditional practice of casting and bringing the patient back to clinic in 10 to 14 days, then removing the cast and obtaining repeat radiographs cost $677. The expense would be much greater if a diagnosis was not made at the time of follow-up, because a routine MR imaging examination was often eventually obtained if a clinical suspicion for a scaphoid fracture remained. Dorsay and colleagues[17] also suggested that lost productivity costs for patients who are

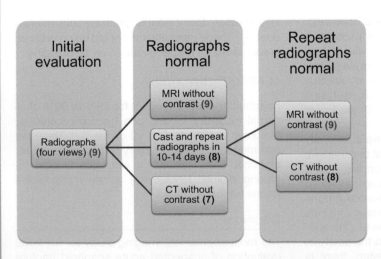

Fig. 3. American College of Radiology (ACR) Appropriateness Criteria (AC) for the evaluation of a suspected acute scaphoid fracture. The numbers following the modalities in parentheses refer to the ACR AC rating scale[1–9]: 1, 2, and 3 are usually not appropriate; 4, 5, and 6 may be appropriate; 7, 8, and 9 are usually appropriate. The most appropriate imaging study for the initial evaluation of the acute suspected scaphoid fracture is radiography, consisting of 4 views including posteroanterior (PA), lateral, semipronated oblique, and PA with ulnar deviation. If the initial radiographs are normal, noncontrast MR imaging is the next most appropriate imaging modality (AC rating 9). Other options at this time are casting and repeat radiography in 10 to 14 days (AC rating 8) and noncontrast CT (AC rating 7). If MR imaging or CT was not available or casting was chosen as a treatment option, repeat radiographs are taken 10 to 14 days later. If the repeat radiographs show negative results, noncontrast MR imaging is the next most appropriate imaging modality (AC rating 9), followed by noncontrast CT (AC rating 8).

potentially unnecessarily immobilized may be great. Similar cost-effectiveness results have been shown in other non-US studies with inference of substantial productivity loss.[1,18–21] Early MR imaging can also provide alternative diagnoses when a scaphoid fracture is not present.[1,22]

The rationale behind casting and repeating the radiographs in 10 to 14 days is that resorptive changes about the fracture make it more conspicuous during 1 to 2 weeks.[23] This practice has been widely accepted and used throughout the world; however, it suffers from poor interobserver reliability (κ = 0.18–0.53).[24,25] The most important potential consequence of casting and waiting for 10 to 14 days is a missed fracture that may require surgical intervention, which could result in an increased incidence of complications, decreased quality of life, and increased costs. If the decision was made to apply cast to the patient following the initial negative results on radiographs and the repeat radiographs in 10 to 14 days also show negative results, the most appropriate imaging options are noncontrast MR imaging (AC rating 9) and noncontrast CT (AC rating 8) (see **Fig. 3**).[2] Noncontrast MR imaging once again is the most appropriate examination for all of the reasons previously discussed. If there are contraindications to MR imaging (eg, claustrophobia, metallic foreign body in the orbit), CT provides a good alternative. In a large meta-analysis including 10 MR imaging and 6 CT studies, with most using follow-up radiographs as the reference standard, there were comparable sensitivities and specificities between the modalities, with MR imaging slightly outperforming CT (MR imaging: sensitivity 96%, specificity 99%; CT: sensitivity 93%, specificity 99%).[26] About 50% of CT studies did not report the time from injury to the imaging examination. Because resorptive changes about the fracture increase with time and CT has a greater sensitivity than radiography for these changes, CT sensitivity would be expected to increase with time, whereas MR imaging is highest immediately after injury. MR imaging is favored over CT at this point in the workup because it not only does not impart any ionizing radiation but also can provide alternative diagnoses as mentioned earlier.

Osteonecrosis

Scaphoid nonunion can lead to osteonecrosis. The retrograde nature of the blood supply to the scaphoid, from the dorsal branch of the radial artery, plays a key role in the incidence of scaphoid osteonecrosis and depends on the location of the fracture. Fractures of the distal pole of the scaphoid have a better prognosis than

fractures of the proximal pole because of this blood supply.[27] The incidence of osteonecrosis is 30% when the fracture involves the middle third of the scaphoid.[28,29] When the fracture involves the proximal one-fifth, the incidence jumps to 100%.[28,29] The viability of the proximal fragment determines whether a nonvascularized or vascularized bone graft is used. In cases in which the proximal pole is found to have a poor blood supply, a vascularized bone graft is preferred with good results.[30–32]

MR imaging is the imaging modality of choice to assess viability of the proximal fragment in scaphoid nonunion.[33–38] However, the most efficacious MR imaging protocol for this purpose is not universally agreed upon. Imaging of scaphoid nonunion may be performed without and with intravenous gadolinium. After the administration of intravenous gadolinium, images can be acquired in a delayed fashion at a single time point or dynamically over multiple early time points to generate a perfusion curve.

A few studies have shown that delayed contrast-enhanced MR imaging examinations can predict the viability of the proximal pole fragment of a scaphoid nonunion better than a non–contrast-enhanced examination when surgical punctate bleeding points of the proximal pole are used as a reference standard.[33,34] One study directly compared delayed contrast-enhanced MR imaging with dynamic contrast-enhanced MR imaging and found that delayed contrast-enhanced MR imaging was superior to dynamic contrast-enhanced MR imaging, which often did not correlate with histopathology.[35] However, Ng and colleagues[38] found no statistical difference between noncontrast, delayed contrast-enhanced, and dynamic contrast-enhanced MR imaging in assessing the proximal pole vascularity, using surgical punctate bleeding as a reference standard.

Two groups studied noncontrast T1-weighted images for the assessment of proximal fragment viability in scaphoid nonunion. Anderson and colleagues[37] compared noncontrast T1-weighted images with delayed contrast-enhanced T1-weighted fat-saturated images. They found poor correlation of the delayed contrast-enhanced images with the intraoperative findings of osteonecrosis; 6 of the 13 patients with intraoperative findings of osteonecrosis had contrast enhancement of the proximal pole, suggesting vascularity (54% sensitivity). These same patients also demonstrated confluent decreased T1 signal of the proximal fragment on the noncontrast images, which correctly identified osteonecrosis (100% sensitivity).[37] Fox and colleagues[36] placed their patients in a moderate- to high-risk category for osteonecrosis if the proximal pole fragment demonstrated confluent decreased

T1 signal on the noncontrast images. They concluded that noncontrast T1-weighted images were comparable to delayed contrast-enhanced MR imaging with similar sensitivities, specificities, and accuracy (54%, 94%, and 79%, respectively).[36]

Based on the current literature, the most appropriate imaging protocol to assess viability of the proximal fragment in scaphoid nonunion is debatable. It is unclear why there are discrepant results in the studies conducted, but there are some theories that may help explain some of the inconsistencies and confounding results.

Reference standards (applies to noncontrast and contrast-enhanced magnetic resonance imaging)
In the vast majority of papers, observation of intraoperative surgical punctate bleeding points at the debrided fracture margins is considered the reference standard in assessing the viability/perfusion of the bone. Unfortunately, this reference standard may not be entirely reliable and accurate for diagnosing osteonecrosis.[39] Histopathologic findings of osteonecrosis are often patchy and can coexist in direct apposition with viable bone,[40] resulting in sampling error when random biopsies are taken, introducing a degree of uncertainty in the reference standard.

Preserved T1 marrow signal (applies to noncontrast magnetic resonance imaging)
As discussed before, the presence of confluent decreased T1 marrow signal is associated with osteonecrosis of the proximal fragment.[36,37] Conversely, the preservation of the normal fat signal should represent viable bone. However,

when avascular necrosis occurs in the femoral head, the central necrotic region maintains bright T1 fat signal because of the presence of fatty acids from hydrolyzed triglycerides.[33,41,42] This same process is postulated to occur in the scaphoid, although the true incidence is not known, and the well demarcated inflammatory tissue at the interface between necrotic and viable bone is not typically seen (**Fig. 4**).[33,38]

Contrast enhancement of the proximal pole (applies to delayed contrast-enhanced magnetic resonance imaging)
Contrast enhancement of the proximal fragment on delayed contrast-enhanced MR imaging does not necessarily connote preserved vascularity. Two theories have been proposed to explain why an osteonecrotic proximal fragment enhances, contrast diffusion across the fracture nonunion and fibrous tissue ingrowth about the fracture. On delayed contrast-enhanced MR imaging, the images are typically acquired 4 to 9 minutes after the administration of intravenous gadolinium.[36,43] This time is sufficient to potentially allow contrast diffusion across the fracture, producing a false-positive result.[36,43] In addition, the presence of fibrous tissue, which can occur as part of a healing response, may enhance, also resulting in a false-positive result.[36,41]

Time of magnetic resonance imaging from injury (applies to dynamic contrast-enhanced magnetic resonance imaging)
Ng and colleagues[38] discovered in a small subset of patients that the time between injury and

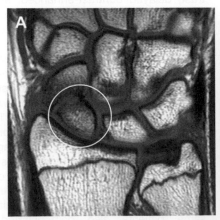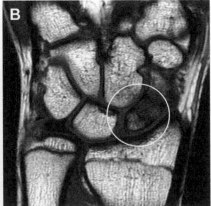

Fig. 4. Noncontrast T1-weighted images used to assess for proximal pole viability in scaphoid nonunion. (*A*) Near-complete preservation of the T1 marrow signal within the proximal pole of the scaphoid nonunion (*circle*). However, at the time of surgery, there was no punctate bleeding identified at the fracture margin of the proximal pole. Therefore, the proximal pole fragment was considered nonviable and a vascularized bone graft was done. (*B*) Patchy T1 marrow signal preservation within the proximal pole of another scaphoid nonunion (*circle*). At the time of surgery, punctate bleeding was identified at the fracture margin of the proximal pole, which was considered viable, and a nonvascularized bone graft was done.

contrast-enhanced MR imaging may play a role in the ability of MR imaging to assess the viability of the proximal fragment. In the 5 indeterminate cases, the average time from injury to MR imaging was long, 101 months.[38] Enhancement of the proximal scaphoid fragment was compared with that of the distal fragment. In these 5 cases, the dynamic enhancement slope was flat in both the distal and proximal fragments, a finding that would typically suggest fair to poor vascularity, but this was not the case at surgery.[38] They concluded that caution must be taken in interpreting the enhancement curve of the proximal fragment when the slope of the distal fragment was also flat, which may be related to the length of time from injury.[38]

Example case

A 34-year-old male right-hand-dominant laboratory worker presented to the Hand Surgery Clinic complaining of chronic right wrist pain. Five years earlier, he had fallen onto his outstretched right hand but did not seek appropriate medical attention. His radiographs demonstrated a chronic un-united scaphoid waist fracture without findings for proximal pole sclerosis, fragmentation, collapse, or secondary degenerative arthritis at the radioscaphoid articulation (**Fig. 5**A, B). This finding, along with his clinical presentation, was consistent with the diagnosis of a scaphoid nonunion. To assist in surgical planning, viability of the proximal pole of the scaphoid was assessed using dynamic contrast-enhanced MR imaging. The noncontrast portion of the MR imaging demonstrated complete preservation of the T1 marrow signal of the proximal pole fragment without increased T2 signal (see **Fig. 5**C, D), suggesting a viable proximal pole fragment. The T2/short tau inversion recovery signal is not typically helpful in the assessment of osteonecrosis according to the authors' experience and the literature.[33,36,37] At the authors' institution, dynamic contrast enhancement is used in a supplemental fashion and not interpreted in isolation. The dynamic contrast-enhanced portion of the examination demonstrated that the proximal pole fragment of the scaphoid had a similar contrast enhancement curve to that of the adjacent, unaffected capitate, suggesting viability (see **Fig. 5**E, F). At the first minute, the contrast enhancement curves show essentially identical relative intensity units indicating rapid, equal contrast enhancement (see **Fig. 5**F). Based on these findings suggesting viability of the proximal pole, the decision was made to treat the scaphoid nonunion with a nonvascularized iliac crest autograft. At the time of surgery, the proximal scaphoid fragment was found to have punctate bleeding points with the tourniquet down after freshening the fracture margins, compatible with viability (see **Fig. 5**G). After 5 months, the nonunion was healed with solid incorporation of the nonvascularized bone graft (see **Fig. 5**H).

OTHER CARPAL FRACTURES

The remaining carpal bones account for 11% to 42% of carpal fractures, with the triquetrum and hamate being the most commonly affected.[7–9,44] The latter carpal fractures account for 4% to 10% of injuries identified in the workup of suspected, radiographically occult, scaphoid fractures.[1,20] Fractures of the triquetrum and hamate are discussed further as they are the next most common carpal fractures. MR imaging can be particularly useful in children with suspected carpal injuries in whom the carpal bones may not all be ossified and therefore not visible on radiography.[45] Although the cartilaginous portions of these immature carpal bones can be seen with ultrasonography and CT, the ability to assess for edema related to injury is limited when compared with MR imaging.

Triquetrum

The most common triquetral fracture pattern is one that involves the dorsal cortex.[46–51] Dorsal triquetral fractures can occur with a fall forward onto a palmar flexed hand or backward onto a dorsiflexed hand.[46–49] There are 2 leading theories regarding the cause of dorsal triquetral fractures. One theory suggests that the fracture results as an avulsion injury from dorsal capsular ligaments,[46,47] whereas the other suggests that the fracture is a result of a chisel action caused by an elongated ulnar styloid process.[48,49] The ligaments that attach to the dorsal triquetrum are discussed in detail elsewhere in this issue. These ligaments include the extrinsic (dorsal radiocarpal and dorsal ulnotriquetral) and intrinsic (dorsal intercarpal) ligaments, each with separate attachment points. Dorsal triquetral fractures can rarely lead to nonunion[51]; however, they are frequently associated with ligament injuries, which can lead to instability and early arthritis.[50,51]

For acute wrist injuries, the ACR AC recommend radiography as the initial imaging modality.[2] As discussed with scaphoid fractures, the initial radiographs may not allow detection of this particular carpal fracture. In the event of unrevealing initial radiographs and a difficult or confounding clinical examination, early MR imaging would be a good choice, as it is the only modality that can confidently provide the appropriate diagnosis

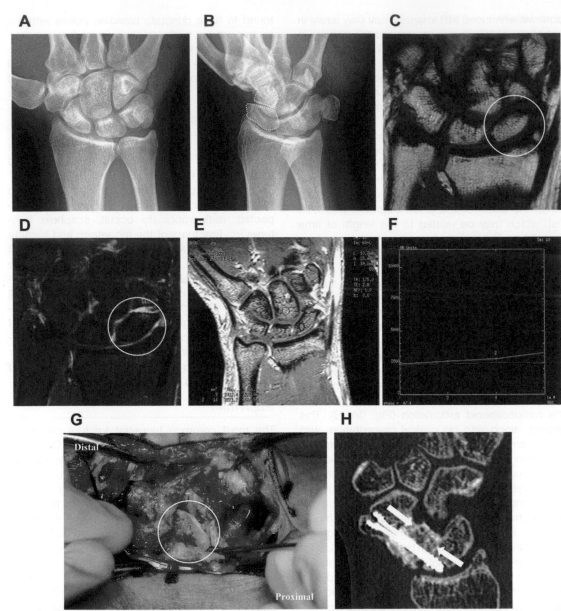

Fig. 5. A 34-year-old man presented to the Hand Surgery Clinic complaining of chronic right wrist pain. Five years earlier, he had fallen onto his outstretched right hand but did not seek appropriate medical attention. (*A, B*) PA and oblique radiographs demonstrate a chronic un-united scaphoid waist fracture (*B*, dotted outline surrounding the distal and proximal fragments) without proximal pole sclerosis, fragmentation, collapse, or secondary degenerative arthritis at the radioscaphoid articulation. Noncontrast coronal MR imaging demonstrates complete preservation of the T1 marrow signal of the proximal pole fragment (*C*, circle) without increased T2 signal (*D*, circle), compatible with proximal pole viability at the authors' institution. (*E*) Coronal dynamic contrast-enhanced non-fat suppressed T1-weighted image illustrating the regions of interest (ROI). A purple ROI is placed over the proximal scaphoid pole and is compared with the green ROI placed over the nearby unaffected capitate. (*F*) Nearly identical dynamic contrast enhancement curves of the proximal scaphoid fragment and the capitate, supportive of viability of the proximal scaphoid pole (x-axis, minutes; y-axis, relative MR contrast units). (*G*) Intraoperative photograph showing the punctate bleeding at the proximal scaphoid fracture margin (*circle*) with the tourniquet deflated. (*H*) Noncontrast sagittal oblique CT of the scaphoid 5 months after nonvascularized iliac crest bone graft with headless screw fixation. There is solid bridging bone across the prior nonunion at the graft interfaces (*arrows*).

and evaluate for a concomitant ligament injury at the same time (**Fig. 6**). There are no comparative studies to date that have evaluated the diagnostic utility and feasibility of MR imaging in the early evaluation of dorsal triquetral fractures.

Hamate

Hamate fractures can involve the body and the hook, with hook fractures being more common.[52] Hook of the hamate fractures are seen in racquet sports, baseball, and golf, with mechanisms of injury that include direct compression and repetitive microtrauma.[51,53,54]

Again, for acute wrist injuries, the ACR AC recommend radiography as the initial imaging modality.[2] If the initial radiographs show normal findings, and a hook of the hamate fracture is suspected, an additional carpal tunnel view is appropriate (AC rating 9) (**Fig. 7**). Standard radiography, without a carpal tunnel view, has been shown to identify only 31% of hamate hook fractures in patients, when using CT as a reference standard.[55] Klausmeyer and Mudgal[53] analyzed

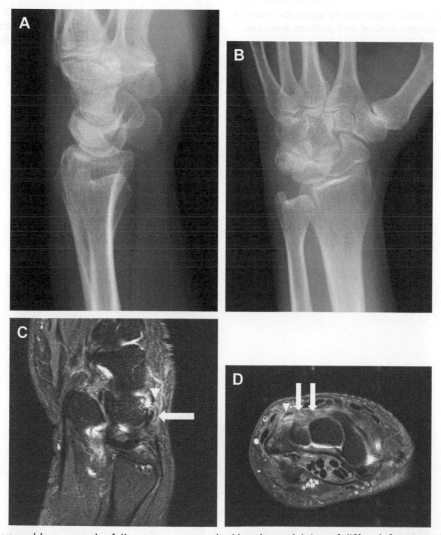

Fig. 6. A 59-year-old woman who fell onto an outstretched hand complaining of diffuse left wrist pain. Negative results on initial radiographs (lateral (*A*) and semipronated oblique (*B*) only shown). Early MR imaging of the wrist was performed 2 days after initial radiography. (*C*) Sagittal T2-weighted fat-saturated MR image demonstrating a dorsal triquetral fracture (*arrowhead*), which remains attached to the dorsal intercarpal ligament. There is increased T2 signal and thickening of the triquetral attachment of the dorsal radiocarpal ligament consistent with a partial tear (*arrow*). (*D*) Axial T2-weighted fat-saturated MR image shows the dorsal intercarpal ligament, radial to the dorsal cortical fracture fragment (*arrowhead*), which is indistinct and demonstrates increased T2 signal also compatible with a partial tear (*arrows*).

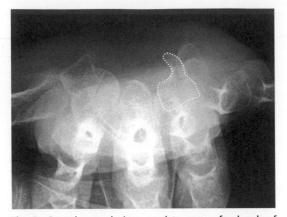

Fig. 7. Carpal tunnel view used to assess for hook of the hamate (*dotted outline*) and pisiform fractures.

prior studies that used the carpal tunnel view for diagnosis of a hook of the hamate fracture and found an overall sensitivity of 40% to 50%, also using CT as the reference standard. Early diagnosis and treatment of hamate hook fractures is important to minimize the risks of complications, including nonunion, flexor digitorum profundus tendon ruptures, ulnar neuritis, and ulnar artery injury.[51,56] Given the poor sensitivity of radiography in the diagnosis of hook of the hamate fractures, noncontrast CT (AC rating 9) and noncontrast MR imaging (AC rating 5) should be considered.[2] MR imaging is the only modality that can both diagnose a hook of the hamate fracture and simultaneously evaluate for all of its potential complications (**Fig. 8**). As with dorsal triquetral fractures, there are no published studies

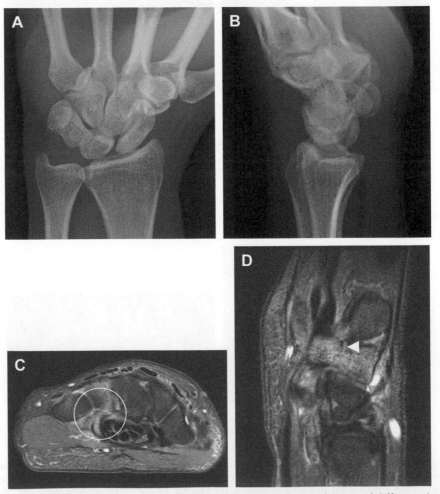

Fig. 8. A 36-year-old woman who fell onto her outstretched left hand, complaining of diffuse wrist pain. Negative results were seen on initial radiographs (PA [*A*] and lateral [*B*] only shown). Early MR imaging of the wrist was performed after initial radiography. (*C*) Axial T2-weighted fat-saturated MR image demonstrating a minimally displaced fracture through the base of the hook of the hamate with surrounding bone marrow edema (*circle*). (*D*) Sagittal T2-weighted fat-saturated MR image also shows the hook of the hamate fracture (*arrowhead*).

that have evaluated the diagnostic utility and feasibility of MR imaging in the early evaluation of hook of the hamate fractures.

SUMMARY

Timely diagnosis of carpal fractures is important for optimal treatment outcome. MR imaging performed early in the workup can provide an accurate and specific diagnosis, as well as uncover developing complications. In the absence of carpal fractures, MR imaging can provide alternative diagnoses such as other unsuspected fractures involving the distal radius/ulna or hand, osseous contusions, and soft-tissue injuries to various ligaments about the wrist. Although MR imaging is the imaging modality of choice to assess the viability of the proximal fragment in scaphoid nonunion, the optimal imaging protocol is not universally agreed upon.

REFERENCES

1. Tibrewal S, Jayakumar P, Vaidya S, et al. Role of MRI in the diagnosis and management of patients with clinical scaphoid fracture. Int Orthop 2012;36(1):107–10.
2. American College of Radiology. ACR appropriateness criteria: acute hand and wrist trauma rev. 2013. Available at: https://acsearch.acr.org/docs/69418/Narrative/.
3. Mettler FA, Huda W, Yoshizumi TT, et al. Effective doses in radiology and diagnostic nuclear medicine: a catalog. Radiology 2008;248(1):254–63.
4. Thavarajah D, Syed T, Shah Y, et al. Does scaphoid bone bruising lead to occult fracture? A prospective study of 50 patients. Injury 2011;42(11):1303–6.
5. La Hei N, McFadyen I, Brock M, et al. Scaphoid bone bruising–probably not the precursor of asymptomatic non-union of the scaphoid. J Hand Surg Eur Vol 2007;32(3):337–40.
6. Brinckman MA, Chau C, Ross JS. Marrow edema variability in acute spine fractures. Spine J 2014. http://dx.doi.org/10.1016/j.spinee.2014.09.032.
7. Hey HW, Chong AK, Murphy D. Prevalence of carpal fracture in Singapore. J Hand Surg Am 2011;36(2):278–83.
8. Hove LM. Fractures of the hand. Distribution and relative incidence. Scand J Plast Reconstr Surg Hand Surg 1993;27:317–9.
9. van Onselen EB, Karim RB, Hage JJ, et al. Prevalence and distribution of hand fractures. J Hand Surg Br 2003;28(5):491–5.
10. Green DP, Hotchkiss RN, Pederson WC, et al. Green's operative hand surgery. Philadelphia: Elsevier/Churchill Livingstone; 2011. p. 639.
11. Herbert TJ, Fisher WE. Management of the fractured scaphoid using a new bone screw. J Bone Joint Surg Br 1984;66B:114–23.
12. Steinmann SP, Adams JE. Scaphoid fractures and non-unions: diagnosis and treatment. J Orthop Sci 2006;11:424–31.
13. Hunter JC, Escobedo EM, Wilson AJ, et al. MR imaging of clinically suspected scaphoid fractures. AJR Am J Roentgenol 1997;168(5):1287–93.
14. Breitenseher MJ, Trattnig S, Gäbler C, et al. MRI in radiologically occult scaphoid fractures. Initial experiences with 1.0 tesla (whole body-middle field equipment) versus 0.2 tesla (dedicated low-field equipment). Radiologe 1997;37(10):812–8 [in German].
15. Gaebler C, Kukla C, Breitenseher M, et al. Magnetic resonance imaging of occult scaphoid fractures. J Trauma 1996;41(1):73–6.
16. Bretlau T, Christensen OM, Edström P, et al. Diagnosis of scaphoid fracture and dedicated extremity MRI. Acta Orthop Scand 1999;70(5):504–8.
17. Dorsay TA, Major NM, Helms CA. Cost-effectiveness of immediate MR imaging versus traditional follow-up for revealing radiographically occult scaphoid fractures. AJR Am J Roentgenol 2001;177(6):1257–63.
18. Gooding A, Coates M, Rothwell A, Accident Compensation Corporation. Cost analysis of traditional follow-up protocol versus MRI for radiographically occult scaphoid fractures: a pilot study for the Accident Compensation Corporation. N Z Med J 2004;117(1201):U1049.
19. Brooks S, Cicuttini FM, Lim S, et al. Cost-effectiveness of adding magnetic resonance imaging to the usual management of suspected scaphoid fractures. Br J Sports Med 2005;39(2):75–9.
20. Brydie A, Raby N. Early MRI in the management of clinical scaphoid fracture. Br J Radiol 2003;76(905):296–300.
21. Patel NK, Davies N, Mirza Z, et al. Cost and clinical effectiveness of MRI in occult scaphoid fractures: a randomised controlled trial. Emerg Med J 2013;30(3):202–7.
22. Kirkeby L, Kairelyte V, Hansen TB. Early magnetic resonance imaging in patients with a clinically suspected scaphoid fracture may identify occult wrist injuries. J Hand Surg Eur Vol 2013;38(5):571–2.
23. Munk PL, Lee MJ, Logan PM, et al. Scaphoid bone waist fractures, acute and chronic: imaging with different techniques. AJR Am J Roentgenol 1997;168(3):779–86.
24. Tiel-van Buul MM, van Beek EJ, Broekhuizen AH, et al. Diagnosing scaphoid fractures: radiographs cannot be used as a gold standard! Injury 1992;23(2):77–9.
25. Low G, Raby N. Can follow-up radiography for acute scaphoid fracture still be considered a valid investigation? Clin Radiol 2005;60(10):1106–10.
26. Yin ZG, Zhang JB, Kan SL, et al. Diagnosing suspected scaphoid fractures: a systematic review

and meta-analysis. Clin Orthop Relat Res 2010; 468(3):723–34.

27. Gelberman RH, Menon J. The vascularity of the scaphoid bone. J Hand Surg Am 1980;5(5):508–13.

28. Cooney WP, Dobyns JH, Linscheid RL. Fractures of the scaphoid: a rational approach to management. Clin Orthop Relat Res 1980;149:90–7.

29. Inoue G, Sakuma M. The natural history of scaphoid non-union. Radiographical and clinical analysis in 102 cases. Arch Orthop Trauma Surg 1996;115(1):1–4.

30. Kawamura K, Chung KC. Treatment of scaphoid fractures and non-unions. J Hand Surg Am 2008; 33(6):988–97.

31. Waitayawinyu T, McCallister WV, Katolik LI, et al. Outcome after vascularized bone grafting of scaphoid non-unions with avascular necrosis. J Hand Surg Am 2009;34(3):387–94.

32. Sunagawa T, Bishop AT, Muramatsu K. Role of conventional and vascularized bone grafts in scaphoid non-union with avascular necrosis: a canine experimental study. J Hand Surg Am 2000;25(5):849–59.

33. Cerezal L, Abascal F, Canga A, et al. Usefulness of gadolinium-enhanced MR imaging in the evaluation of the vascularity of scaphoid non-unions. AJR Am J Roentgenol 2000;174(1):141–9.

34. Schmitt R, Christopoulos G, Wagner M, et al. Avascular necrosis (AVN) of the proximal fragment in scaphoid non-union: is intravenous contrast agent necessary in MRI? Eur J Radiol 2011;77(2):222–7.

35. Donati OF, Zanetti M, Nagy L, et al. Is dynamic gadolinium enhancement needed in MR imaging for the preoperative assessment of scaphoidal viability in patients with scaphoid non-union? Radiology 2011; 260(3):808–16.

36. Fox MG, Gaskin CM, Chhabra AB, et al. Assessment of scaphoid viability with MRI: a reassessment of findings on unenhanced MR images. AJR Am J Roentgenol 2010;195(4):W281–6.

37. Anderson SE, Steinbach LS, Tschering-Vogel D, et al. MR imaging of avascular scaphoid non-union before and after vascularized bone grafting. Skeletal Radiol 2005;34(6):314–20.

38. Ng AW, Griffith JF, Taljanovic MS, et al. Is dynamic contrast-enhanced MRI useful for assessing proximal fragment vascularity in scaphoid fracture delayed and non-union? Skeletal Radiol 2013;42(7): 983–92.

39. Green DP. The effect of avascular necrosis on Russe bone grafting for scaphoid non-union. J Hand Surg Am 1985;10(5):597–605.

40. Urban MA, Green DP, Aufdemorte TB. The patchy configuration of scaphoid avascular necrosis. J Hand Surg Am 1993;18(4):669–74.

41. Sakai T, Sugano N, Nishii T, et al. MR findings of necrotic lesions and the extralesional area of osteonecrosis of the femoral head. Skeletal Radiol 2000; 29(3):133–41.

42. Vande Berg B, Malghem J, Labaisse MA, et al. Avascular necrosis of the hip: comparison of contrast-enhanced and nonenhanced MR imaging with histologic correlation. Work in progress. Radiology 1992;182(2):445–50.

43. Sebag G, Ducou Le Pointe H, Klein I, et al. Dynamic gadolinium-enhanced subtraction MR imaging–a simple technique for the early diagnosis of Legg-Calvé-Perthes disease: preliminary results. Pediatr Radiol 1997;27(3):216–20.

44. Raghupathi AK, Kumar P. Nonscaphoid carpal injuries - incidence and associated injuries. J Orthop 2014;11(2):91–5.

45. Obdeijn MC, van der Vlies CH, van Rijn RR. Capitate and hamate fracture in a child: the value of MRI imaging. Emerg Radiol 2010;17(2):157–9.

46. Bonnin JG, Greening WP. Fractures of the triquetrum. Br J Surg 1944;31:278–83.

47. Smith DK, Murray PM. Avulsion fractures of the volar aspect of triquetral bone of the wrist: a subtle sign of carpal ligament injury. AJR Am J Roentgenol 1996; 166:609–14.

48. Levy M, Fischel RE, Stern GM, et al. Chip fractures of the os triquetrum: the mechanism of injury. J Bone Joint Surg Br 1979;61:355–7.

49. Garcia-Elias M. Dorsal fractures of the triquetrum-avulsion or compression fractures? J Hand Surg Am 1987;12(2):266–8.

50. Becce F, Theumann N, Bollmann C, et al. Dorsal fractures of the triquetrum: MRI findings with an emphasis on dorsal carpal ligament injuries. AJR Am J Roentgenol 2013;200(3):608–17 [Erratum appears in AJR Am J Roentgenol 2013;201(3):698].

51. Suh N, Ek ET, Wolfe SW. Carpal fractures. J Hand Surg Am 2014;39(4):785–91 [quiz: 791].

52. Milch H. Fracture of the hamate bone. J Bone Joint Surg Am 1932;16:459–62.

53. Klausmeyer MA, Mudgal CS. Hook of hamate fractures. J Hand Surg Am 2013;38(12):2457–60 [quiz: 2460].

54. Vigler M, Aviles A, Lee SK. Carpal fractures excluding the scaphoid [Review]. Hand Clin 2006; 22(4):501–16 [abstract: vii].

55. Kato H, Nakamura R, Horii E, et al. Diagnostic imaging for fracture of the hook of the hamate. Hand Surg 2000;5(1):19–24.

56. O'Shea K, Weiland AJ. Fractures of the hamate and pisiform bones. Hand Clin 2012;28(3):287–300, viii.

Imaging of the Proximal and Distal Radioulnar Joints

Eric C. Ehman, MD[a],*, Joel P. Felmlee, PhD[b],
Matthew A. Frick, MD[b]

KEYWORDS

- Radius • Ulna • Wrist • Elbow • CT • MR imaging • Radiology

KEY POINTS

- The proximal radioulnar joint (PRUJ) and distal radioulnar joint (DRUJ) are complex joints; diagnosis of pathologic abnormality requires an understanding of not only anatomy but also the relevant biomechanics.
- Radiography forms the initial evaluation of both joints.
- Computed tomography (CT) is useful for the evaluation of bony structures and can provide 3-dimensional modeling of complex abnormalities, such as fractures.
- MR imaging should be obtained when soft tissue such as ligamentous, muscular, or tendinous pathologic abnormality is suspected.
- Particularly in the evaluation of the DRUJ, knowledge of the patient's operative history and findings on physical examination are important to tailor protocols such as dynamic CT to extract maximal benefit.

ROTATIONAL MOTION OF THE FOREARM ALLOWS 3-DIMENSIONAL POSITIONING OF THE HAND IN SPACE

The PRUJ and DRUJ form the proximal and distal articulations between the radius and the ulna, a unique skeletal arrangement, which, along with the interosseous membrane, allows for the 150° pivot motion of the forearm from pronation to supination, positioning the hand in space, and enabling a wide variety of tasks.

Derangements of the DRUJ and PRUJ may occur secondary to trauma to the hand, wrist, forearm, or elbow, in the setting of degenerative or overuse injuries or within the context of inflammatory or crystalline arthropathies.

Evaluation of these dynamic joints is challenging for hand surgeons and radiologists alike due not only to the structural relationships but also to the functional interaction between the various bones, muscles, and ligaments.

ANATOMY AND BIOMECHANICS
Proximal Radioulnar Joint

The PRUJ is a synovial pivot joint formed by the interface between the cylindrical radial head and the radial notch of the ulna (**Fig. 1**). Motion at the

Disclosures: Dr Ehman EC: none; Dr Felmlee has intellectual property rights and a financial interest in the BC10 wrist coil; Dr Frick MA: none.
[a] Department of Radiology and Biomedical Imaging, University of California, San Francisco, 505 Parnassus Avenue, San Francisco, CA 94143, USA; [b] Department of Radiology, Mayo Clinic, 200 First Street SW, Rochester, MN 55905, USA
* Corresponding author.
E-mail address: eric.ehman@ucsf.edu

Magn Reson Imaging Clin N Am 23 (2015) 417–425
http://dx.doi.org/10.1016/j.mric.2015.04.011
1064-9689/15/$ – see front matter © 2015 Elsevier Inc. All rights reserved.

mri.theclinics.com

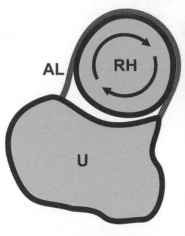
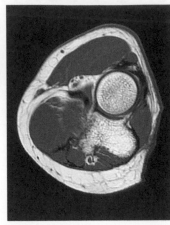

Fig. 1. Axial diagram of the left PRUJ (*left*) and T1-weighted axial MR image (*right*) depicting the position of the radial head (RH) within the radial notch of the proximal ulna (U). The annual ligament (AL) prevents side-to-side translation of the radial head, allowing rotation only (*arrows*). The position of the radial head abutting the capitellum proximally prevents proximal translation.

joint consists of rotation of the radial head. Proximally, pronation is facilitated by the pronator teres, while supination is a result of contraction of the biceps brachii and the supinator muscles. Radial head translation is limited by the annular ligament, which spans the anterior and posterior margins of the radial notch of the ulna, effectively trapping the radial head within. The quadrate ligament is a focal thickening of the inferior annular ligament, which attaches to the radial neck, further anchoring the radius. Support of the annual ligament is provided by attachments to the radial collateral ligament and the joint capsule, which is shared with that of the elbow joint.

Interosseous Membrane

The interosseous membrane, or middle radioulnar joint, is a thin band of fibrous tissue extending from the radius proximally to the ulna distally. This syndesmosis results in attachment of the 2 bones, allowing distribution of forces during loading.[1,2]

Distal Radioulnar Joint

Another synovial pivot joint, the DRUJ, consists of the relationship between the sigmoid notch of the distal radius and the ulnar head (**Fig. 2**). The sigmoid notch of the radius is a hemicylindrical, longitudinally oriented concavity on the ulnar aspect of the distal radius. The adjacent ulnar head is

similarly hemicylindrical, of a smaller radius than the sigmoid notch, however, allowing for anterior and posterior translation as well as rotation of the joint. The head of the ulna subluxes dorsally in pronation and volarly in supination. A third degree of freedom exists, allowing longitudinal translation of the ulna with respect to the radius.[3] The multiple possible axes of translation and rotation introduce an inherent instability of the DRUJ, constrained primarily by tendinous and ligamentous structures.

The ligamentous supporting structures of the DRUJ consist of the dorsal and volar radioulnar ligaments, the ulnocarpal (ulnolunate and ulnotriquetral) ligaments, and the triangular fibrocartilage complex (TFCC), which is anchored to ulnar styloid and the base of the styloid (fovea). The structure, function, and pathology associated with the TFCC are discussed in greater detail in the article Triangular Fibrocartilage Complex by Drs Cody, Nakamura, Small, and Yoshioka.

Additional soft tissue stabilizers are the deep head of the pronator quadratus and the extensor carpi ulnaris. The pronator quadratus provides active approximation of the DRUJ in pronation and passive support in supination. Because of its position overlying the dorsal distal ulna and investment by the extensor retinaculum, the extensor carpi ulnaris subsheath partially stabilizes the DRUJ. Finally, a thin joint capsule provides minimal support.

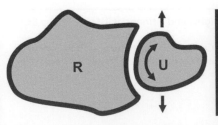
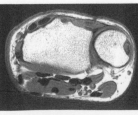

Fig. 2. Axial diagram (*left*) and T1-weighted axial MR image (*right*) of the right DRUJ showing the ulnar head (U) within the sigmoid notch of the distal radius (R). A larger curvature along the sigmoid notch allows for both anterior and posterior translation of the ulnar head as well as rotational motion.

IMAGING ALGORITHMS
Proximal Radioulnar Joint

An imaging algorithm for evaluation of the PRUJ is provided in **Fig. 3**.

Distal Radioulnar Joint

An imaging algorithm for the DRUJ is provided in **Fig. 4**. Note that preimaging knowledge of the wrist examination (stable or unstable) is helpful.

IMAGING OF THE PROXIMAL RADIOULNAR JOINT
Radiography

The PRUJ is typically completely included in standard anteroposterior and lateral views of the elbow, which may demonstrate abnormal alignment of the radial head or fractures of the radial head and the proximal ulna. Dislocation of the radial head is best assessed by comparing the position of the radial head relative to the capitellum rather than the proximal ulna. The radiocapitellar line, a line drawn along the shaft of the proximal radius through the capitellum, should intersect the center of the radial head on both views (**Fig. 5**). If there is displacement of the radial head with respect to this line, dislocation should be considered. Exaggeration of the normally visualized anterior fat pad or the presence of a posterior fat pad on the lateral view indicates an elbow effusion. In the setting of known or suspected trauma, the presence of an elbow effusion without evidence of fracture on the standard radiographic views should prompt additional oblique radiographs or advanced imaging such as CT to exclude an occult fracture.

Computed Tomography

CT is used primarily for the evaluation of bony structures within the PRUJ and may be useful in assessing the articular surfaces of the radial head for cortical step-offs or characterization of comminuted fractures of the radial head (**Fig. 6**).

MR Imaging

MR imaging of the elbow includes the PRUJ and may show cartilage loss related to degenerative

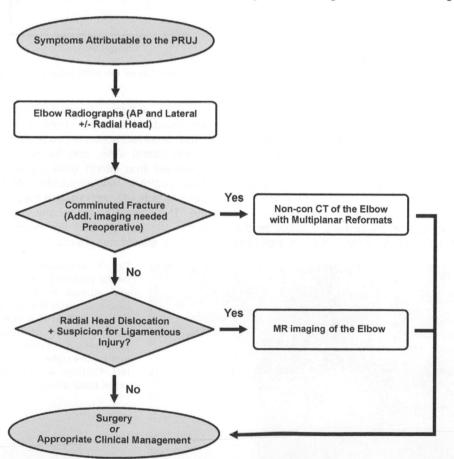

Fig. 3. Imaging algorithm for evaluation of the PRUJ. AP, anteroposterior.

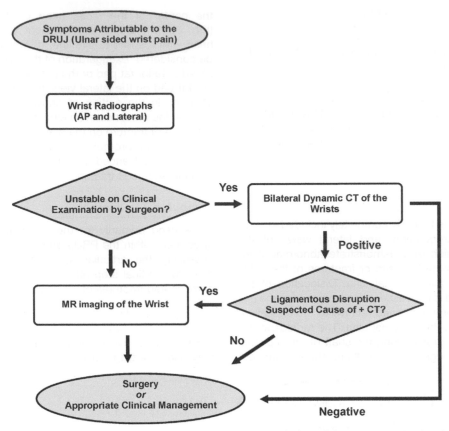

Fig. 4. Imaging algorithm for the DRUJ. Note that preimaging knowledge of the wrist examination (stable or unstable) is helpful.

changes at the radial head or radial notch of the ulna, or discontinuity, thickening, or abnormal signal within the annular ligament suggestive of injury (**Fig. 7**).

IMAGING OF THE DISTAL RADIOULNAR JOINT
Radiography

Plain radiography is the primary modality for the initial evaluation of the wrist and hand, including

the DRUJ.[4] A typical 3-view wrist series may provide valuable information about the integrity of the DRUJ; however, accurate positioning, particularly on the lateral view, can be difficult.[5] A well-positioned true lateral wrist radiograph should show complete superimposition of the lunate, proximal pole of scaphoid, and the proximal capitate. The palmar cortex of the capitate should overlie the pisiform and the distal pole of the scaphoid should not project more anteriorly than

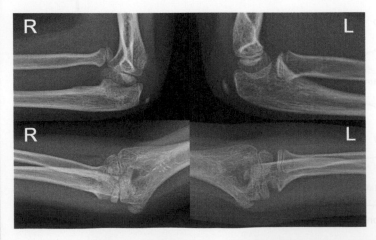

Fig. 5. Anteroposterior (*top*) and lateral (*bottom*) radiographs of bilateral elbows in a 9-year-old with elbow pain and limited range of motion. Note that if a line was drawn along the length of the radial diaphysis, it would not intersect the capitellum on the right, but does so on the left. Findings are consistent with a radial head dislocation.

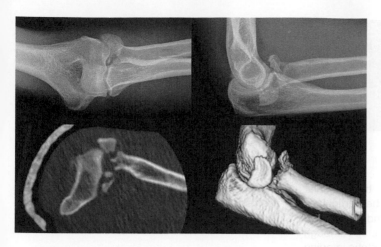

Fig. 6. Anteroposterior and lateral radiographs of the right elbow (*top*) demonstrate a comminuted radial head fracture that is more clearly seen and evaluated at noncontrast CT (*bottom left*). Three-dimensional reformats generated from CT images (*bottom right*) are often useful for operative planning.

the pisiform (**Fig. 8**). On a true lateral radiograph, dorsal or volar subluxation of the ulna with respect to the radius is readily apparent; however, on off-lateral radiographs, subluxation may be underestimated. Because off-lateral radiographs are usually the result of slight supination, apparent dorsal subluxation will be reduced, whereas volar subluxation will be exaggerated.[6,7] Ulnar variance can be accurately measured on neutral posteroanterior (PA) radiographs of the wrist. Other views such as radial- or ulnar-deviated PA radiographs may be useful in evaluation of the wrist but provide minimal additional information regarding the DRUJ.

Computed Tomography

CT is commonly used in the evaluation of the DRUJ.[5,8,9] Able to generate high-resolution images without the use of intravenous contrast in a short period of time, CT is an ideal choice for dynamic imaging of the DRUJ involving acquisition in multiple positions or loadings to confirm clinical suspicion of instability. Routine CT wrist protocols result in a single acquisition through the wrist in a neutral position with the arm above the head (so-called "Superman" or "swimmer's" position). These images are useful for evaluation of trauma to the joint, easily demonstrating fractures, loose

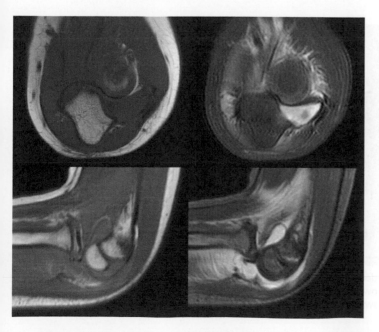

Fig. 7. Axial and sagittal T1-weighted (*left*) and T2-weighed (*right*) images from an MR imaging of the right elbow in a 7-year-old show dislocation of the PRUJ, with trapping of the annual ligament posteriorly, preventing reduction of the dislocation.

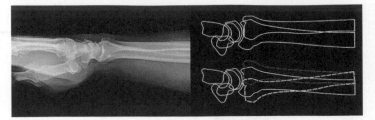

Fig. 8. True lateral radiograph of the wrist (*left*). Note that on outline view (*right*) that the anterior cortex of the capitate overlaps the pisiform and the distal pole of the scaphoid is approximately as far palmar as the pisiform. On lateral view, subluxation of the DRUJ is seen as relative dorsal (*red*) or volar (*green*) displacement of the ulna.

bodies, and the congruence of the articular surfaces. Multiplanar formats may be particularly helpful, and 3-dimensional renderings are frequently favored by surgeons (**Fig. 9**). Although providing excellent anatomic detail, static imaging protocols are limited in evaluation of stress-related changes to joint geometry.

New approaches favor imaging the joint during varying degrees of loading by placing weights on the hand or by use of a dedicated apparatus. In the authors' practice, patients are placed prone on the CT table, with their hands raised above their heads, and they are asked to grip a special set of handles that can be placed in neutral position or directed to fixed pronation or supination. The DRUJ is imaged in each of these 3 positions, followed by active pronation/supination against the grip in each position, resulting in a total of 9 sets of images of each wrist, which are then evaluated for positioning of the ulna with respect to the sigmoid notch (**Fig. 10**).

In the authors' practice, the affected joint is often injected with anesthetic before imaging to prevent false negative studies as a result of patient hesitation to engage in active pronation or supination because of pain or instability.

MR Imaging

MR imaging is often crucial in evaluating pathologic abnormality involving the DRUJ.[10–12] Using tailored sequences and dedicated wrist imaging coils (**Fig. 11**) at 1.5, or preferably, 3.0 T, MR imaging allows direct visualization of ligamentous structures, including the dorsal and volar radioulnar and ulnocarpal ligaments as well as the TFCC including the foveal attachment.

Although rare, tears of the dorsal or volar radioulnar ligaments may be present in patients with a history of trauma. Tears of the TFCC are much more common, and those involving the foveal attachment or avulsion of the ulnar styloid may result in DRUJ instability. The ulnocarpal, particularly the ulnotriquetral, ligaments often result in ulnar-sided wrist pain. With proper technique, each of these structures can be identified at

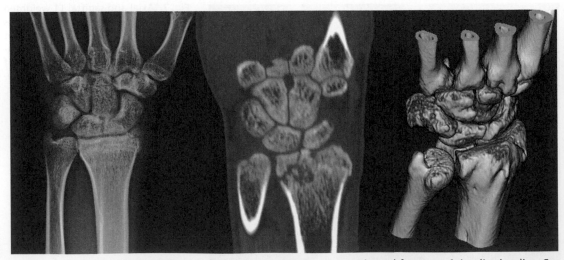

Fig. 9. Left wrist AP radiograph (*left*) demonstrates an impacted, comminuted fracture of the distal radius. Coronal noncontrast CT image (*center*) shows extension in to the DRUJ. Three-dimensional surface-rendering (*right*) generated from CT dataset clearly shows involvement of both the DRUJ and the radiocarpal joint and was requested for surgical planning.

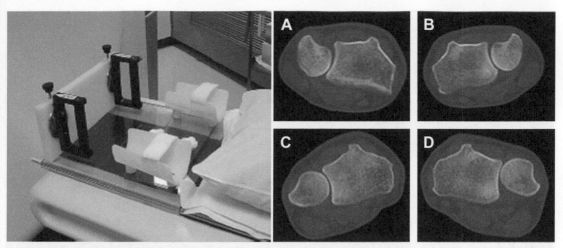

Fig. 10. Device for use with CT for dynamic DRUJ imaging. Axial CT images through both DRUJs (*A*, *C*), right wrist, (*B*, *D*); left wrist shows evidence of subluxation on the left (*D*). (*From* Amrami KK, Moran SL, Berger RA, et al. Imaging the distal radioulnar joint. Hand Clin 2010;26(4):470; with permission.)

routine wrist MR imaging and examined for pathologic abnormality. Although sometimes necessary for evaluation of the more distal wrist, MR arthrography is rarely informative in evaluation of the DRUJ.

Tears of the foveal attachment of the TFCC are one of the most common causes of ulnar-sided wrist pain and DRUJ instability.[13] The foveal attachment is best seen on coronal and sagittal images and appears as a band of low signal intensity that attaches directly to bone in the ulnar fovea. Partial tears may show as abnormal signal within the substance of the ligament. Complete tears may manifest as fluid between the torn remnant and the cortex, best seen on fluid-sensitive sequences such as fat-saturated T2 or short tau inversion recovery (**Fig. 12**). If the wrist is imaged in pronation, complete tears of the dorsal radioulnar ligaments or the foveal attachment of the TFCC may manifest as dorsal subluxation of the ulna with respect to the sigmoid notch, similar to that seen at dynamic CT.[14] Such tears

of the foveal TFCC, either partial or complete, are often associated with ulnotriquetral ligament or the body or disc of the TFCC.

Other sources of ulnar wrist pain including degenerative or inflammatory arthritis of the DRUJ may be best seen at MR imaging. Degenerative arthritis, typically a result of trauma, may present as cartilage loss, subchondral cystic change, or underlying bony injury. In the setting of rheumatoid arthritis and other inflammatory arthropathies, MR imaging is particularly beneficial in demonstrating synovitis of the DRUJ, erosive changes at the ulnar styloid, and possible partial- or full-thickness tears of the foveal attachment of the TFCC.

Postoperative Imaging

Surgical techniques for repair of an unstable DRUJ vary greatly. Routine evaluation typically begins with standard 2-view radiographs of the wrist to evaluate bony relationships and the integrity of

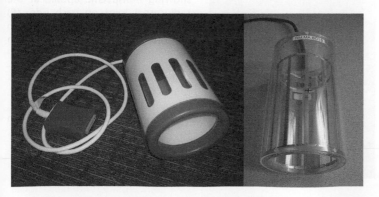

Fig. 11. Dedicated MR receiver coils used for imaging the wrist. US Food and Drug Administration–approved 10-cm birdcage wrist coil (BC-10; Mayo Clinic, Rochester, MN, USA) (*left*) and custom 13-cm birdcage wrist coil (*right*).

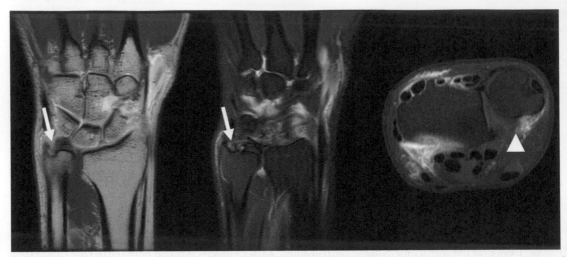

Fig. 12. Coronal T1- (*left*), coronal T2- (*center*), and axial T2-weighted (*right*) images from a 3.0-T MR imaging of the right wrist. On both T1 and T2 images, there is abnormal signal within and discontinuity of the foveal attachment of the TFCC (*arrows*). Also note resulting dorsal subluxation of the ulna with respect to the sigmoid notch of the radius (*arrowhead*).

any implanted devices such as anchors, screws, or prostheses. Cross-sectional imaging is reviewed for cases where repair failure or other complication is suspected. Dynamic CT is helpful for the evaluation for recurrent instability. Metallic artifact from sutures, anchors, and implants may cause image quality degradation secondary to metallic susceptibility artifact. Modification of scanning parameters, such as increasing receiver bandwidth, increasing echo-train length, and use of inversion recovery sequences, in lieu of chemical fat-saturated images help to significantly mitigate these artifacts such that it is usually feasible to acquire diagnostic quality images of the reconstructed DRUJ. Additional recent advances in vendor-specific metallic artifact reduction sequences also show great promise in postoperative

imaging. MR may demonstrate the restoration of normal alignment in pronation and the integrity of muscle or tendon grafts and can reveal complications of pretreatment DRUJ derangement such as early arthritis.

Nuclear Medicine

Scintigraphy may occasionally serve as a useful adjunct to anatomic imaging, specifically when prior anatomic imaging has failed to yield a diagnosis or appropriate differential diagnosis. Radiographs are typically unrevealing in patients with early degenerative or inflammatory arthritis and Technetium-99 bone scan, owing to its high sensitivity, may demonstrate radiographically occult areas of bone turnover or inflammation (**Fig. 13**).

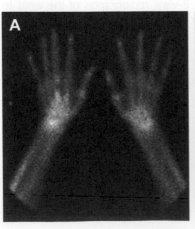
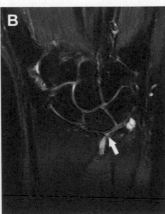

Fig. 13. (*A*) Bone scan from a patient with bilateral ulnar wrist pain showing nonspecific uptake at the radiocarpal joint on each side. (*B*) Coronal T2-weighted fast spin-echo MR image with fat suppression showing the synovitis and radial-sided tear (*arrow*) explaining the activity on the bone scan. (*From* Amrami KK, Moran SL, Berger RA, et al. Imaging the distal radioulnar joint. Hand Clin 2010;26(4):470; with permission.)

In addition, a nuclear medicine whole-body joint scan may also be beneficial in enigmatic cases. Finally, 3-phase bone scans or Indium-111-labeled white blood cell scans may also provide useful diagnostic information when advanced imaging such as MR imaging remains inconclusive.

SUMMARY

The PRUJ and DRUJ are complex joints; diagnosis of pathologic abnormality requires an understanding of not only anatomy but also the relevant biomechanics. Radiography forms the initial evaluation of both joints. CT is useful for evaluation of bony structures and can provide 3-dimensional modeling of complex abnormalities, such as fractures. MR imaging should be obtained when soft tissue, such as ligamentous, muscular, or tendinous, pathologic abnormality is suspected. Particularly in the evaluation of the DRUJ, knowledge of the patient's operative history and findings on physical examination are important to tailor protocols such as dynamic CT to extract maximal benefit.

REFERENCES

1. Wallace AL, Walsh WR, van Rooijen M, et al. The interosseous membrane in radio-ulnar dissociation. J Bone Joint Surg Br 1997;79(3):422–7.
2. Rabinowitz RS, Light TR, Havey RM, et al. The role of the interosseous membrane and triangular fibrocartilage complex in forearm stability. J Hand Surg 1994;19(3):385–93.
3. Palmer AK, Werner FW. Biomechanics of the distal radioulnar joint. Clin Orthop Relat Res 1984;(187): 26–35.
4. Amrami KK, Berger RA. Radiology corner: review of plain radiographs. J Am Soc Surg Hand 2005; 5(1):4–7.
5. Mino DE, Palmer AK, Levinsohn EM. The role of radiography and computerized tomography in the diagnosis of subluxation and dislocation of the distal radioulnar joint. J Hand Surg 1983;8(1):23–31.
6. Kumar A, Iqbal MJ. Missed isolated volar dislocation of distal radio-ulnar joint: a case report. J Emerg Med 1999;17(5):873–5.
7. Zanetti M, Gilula LA, Jacob HA, et al. Palmar tilt of the distal radius: influence of off-lateral projection initial observations 1. Radiology 2001;220(3): 594–600.
8. Tay SC, Berger RA, Tomita K, et al. In vivo three-dimensional displacement of the distal radioulnar joint during resisted forearm rotation. J Hand Surg 2007;32(4):450–8.
9. Nakamura R, Horii E, Imaeda T, et al. Criteria for diagnosing distal radioulnar joint subluxation by computed tomography. Skeletal Radiol 1996;25(7): 649–53.
10. Amrami KK, Moran SL, Berger RA, et al. Imaging the distal radioulnar joint. Hand Clin 2010;26(4):467–75.
11. Amrami KK. Radiology corner: basic principles of MRI for hand surgeons. J Am Soc Surg Hand 2005;5(2):81–6.
12. Amrami KK, Joel PF. 3-Tesla imaging of the wrist and hand: techniques and applications. Semin Musculoskelet Radiol 2008;12(3):223–37.
13. Atzei A, Luchetti R. Foveal TFCC tear classification and treatment. Hand Clin 2011;27(3):263–72.
14. Ehman EC, Hayes ML, Berger RA, et al. Subluxation of the distal radioulnar joint as a predictor of foveal triangular fibrocartilage complex tears. J Hand Surg 2011;36(11):1780–4.

MR Imaging of the Elbow

Daniela Binaghi, MD

KEYWORDS

- MR imaging of the elbow • Elbow anatomy • Elbow instability • Epicondylitis
- Osteochondral injuries of the elbow • Biceps tendon • Triceps tendon

KEY POINTS

- The elbow is a complex anatomic region difficult to assess even by experienced examiners.
- Precise imaging diagnosis helps the management of acute lesions and chronic overuse injuries of the elbow.
- MR imaging is of great importance for patients on the way to regaining a normal elbow joint that permits a functional range of painless motion.

IMAGING PROTOCOLS

MR images are acquired using T1-weighted and T2-weighted and proton density (PD) images, with and without fat suppression. Current protocols differ between specialists, according to their preferences. MR imaging of the elbow is directly dependent on the use of surface coils specialized for the imaging of extremities; moreover, the field of view should be limited to the minimal area necessary to encompass all anatomic structures.

The elbow must be placed close to or at the scanner's isocenter to provide the field homogeneity required for off-center fat suppression. Typically, patients are placed in a supine position with their arm to the side, or in a lateral decubitus position with their back leaning against the scanner. The patient also can be positioned prone with their arm extended overhead (the Superman position), a position that, albeit less well tolerated and more prone to introducing motion degradation artifacts, can be useful with larger patients. In certain situations, such as with biceps insertion pathology, the tendon can be imaged better with the elbow flexed, the shoulder abducted, and the forearm supinated: the so-called FABS (flexed abducted supinated) position.

ANATOMY

The elbow is a complex joint formed by 3 distinct articulations: the ulnohumeral, radiohumeral, and radioulnar articulations. The first 2 articulations function as a hinge, permitting flexion and extension between the arm and forearm; the last 2 accomplish the pivot motion of pronation and supination and are functionally linked to the distal radioulnar joint and the wrist. These joints have a common articular cavity and share a multitude of enveloping structures, including the synovium, capsule, and ligaments, all of which render the elbow a single anatomic unit.

The osseous anatomy of 3 bones: the humerus, radius, and ulna; and, although examining the elbow can appear deceptively simple, knowledge of a few potential MR imaging pitfalls (**Box 1**) can greatly reduce the risk of misdiagnoses, including osteochondral defects (**Figs. 1 and 2**).[1,2]

The capsule of the elbow is reinforced by strong collateral ligaments, but is relatively weak and loose anteriorly and posteriorly, permitting a large range of flexion through extension. The ulnar collateral ligament (UCL) consists of 3 ligamentous bundles (**Fig. 3, Table 1**). The anterior bundle is the major medial stabilizer of the elbow and, fortunately, is the easiest to image (see **Box 1**,

The author has nothing to disclose.
Radiology Department, Favaloro University, Favaloro Foundation, Av Belgrano 1746, Buenos Aires C1093AAS, Argentina
E-mail address: daniela.binaghi@gmail.com

Magn Reson Imaging Clin N Am 23 (2015) 427–440
http://dx.doi.org/10.1016/j.mric.2015.04.005
1064-9689/15/$ – see front matter © 2015 Elsevier Inc. All rights reserved.

Box 1
Anatomic variants that must be recognized and distinguished from pathologic abnormality

Pseudodefect of the capitellum

Pseudolesion of the trochlear notch

The anterior bundle of the UCL and the LUCL frequently have striated appearance

Bifid DBT

Anconeus epitrochlearis

Ulnar nerve high signal intensity on fluid-sensitive sequences[7]

Plicae size less than 3 mm

Figs. 2 and 7). It arises from the medial epicondyle and attaches to the coronoid process (sublime tubercle). This bundle itself has functional anterior and posterior components, with the former component more important in extension and the latter more important in flexion; however, they are not seen as separate structures. The posterior bundle extends from below the medial epicondyle to the medial olecranon, forming the floor of the cubital tunnel. It becomes a secondary stabilizer of the elbow when the joint is flexed beyond 90 . The transverse bundle consists of fibers that extend from the anterior and posterior bundles and does not contribute to elbow stability.[1]

The radial collateral ligament (RCL) is a complex structure (**Fig. 4**, **Table 2**). The annular ligament is the primary stabilizer of the proximal radioulnar joint (PRUJ) and is best seen on axial images wrapping around the side of the radial head from one side of the radial notch to the other. The RCL arises from the anterior margin of the lateral epicondyle, inserts onto the annular ligament and fascia of the supinator muscle, and is best seen on coronal images. The lateral ulnar collateral ligament (LUCL) is the major posterolateral stabilizer and can be seen on coronal or sagittal images, arising more posteriorly and superficially from the lateral epicondyle, and inserting onto the supinator crest.[1,3]

Numerous muscles originate at or insert into the osseous surfaces of the elbow.[4] They can be divided into anterior, posterior, medial, and lateral compartments (**Table 3**).

The distal biceps tendon (DBT) consists of 2 unique anatomic and functional subunits, even though it usually is seen, on imaging, inserting as a single, flat paratenon-lined extrasynovial structure with no tendon sheath (**Fig. 5**). The superficial fibers of the biceps tendon form a broad aponeurotic sheet, termed the lacertus fibrosus (LF), which sweeps across the antecubital fossa, covering and protecting the median nerve and brachial artery. It also blends with the antebrachial fascia that covers the superficial forearm flexors, thereby assisting with forearm supination and elbow flexion. An intact LF can also prevent retraction of a ruptured biceps tendon, facilitating repair of chronic ruptures.[5,6]

The triceps is the only major extensor of the elbow. It is a tripinnate muscle composed of long, lateral, and medial heads. As a result of this

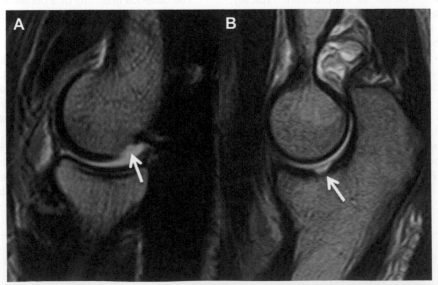

Fig. 1. Anatomic variants to be recognized and distinguished from pathologic abnormality. Sagittal T2-weighted images showing (*A*) pseudodefect of the capitellum (*arrow*); (*B*) pseudolesion of the trochlear notch (*arrow*).

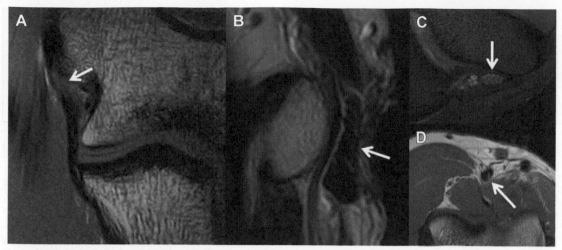

Fig. 2. Anatomic variants to be recognized and distinguished from pathologic abnormality. (*A*) Coronal T1-weighted image shows the typical striated appearance of the UCL (*arrow*). (*B*) Sagittal T2-weighted image demonstrates an anconeus epitrochlearis muscle (*arrow*). (*C*) Axial short tau inversion recovery (STIR) shows the normal appearance of the ulnar nerve at the elbow (*arrow*). (*D*) Axial proton density-weighted image of a bifid DBT (*arrow*).

laminar anatomy, each component may be injured separately. It primarily inserts onto the olecranon and posterior joint capsule.[6]

The 3 major nerves in the elbow are the radial, median, and ulnar nerve. The ulnar nerve is the most frequently injured because it is relatively exposed while coursing through the cubital tunnel; however, ulnar neuropathy may also arise from nontraumatic causes (see **Box 1, Fig. 2**).[7]

The bursae about the elbow joint include the olecranon, bicipitoradial, and interosseous bursae. Bursitis can arise from different causes, with the olecranon bursa the most commonly affected (**Fig. 6**).[8] Several synovial plicae have been described, with the posterolateral plicae being the most frequently identified (see **Box 1, Fig. 6**).[1,2]

ELBOW INSTABILITY

The elbow is one of the most stable articulations in the human skeleton. Because the forces that cross the elbow joint are principally valgus in nature, the joint is not often subjected to varus stress, nor does its articular anatomy predispose it to true varus instability (**Box 2**).

The elbow has both static and dynamic constraints. The 3 primary static constraints are the

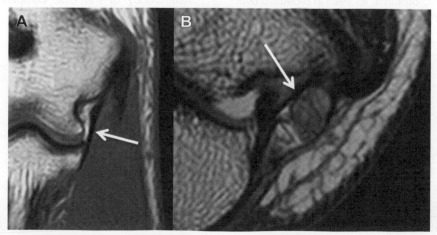

Fig. 3. Normal UCL. (*A*) Coronal T1-weighted image of the anterior bundle (*arrow*). (*B*) Axial PD-weighted image of the posterior bundle (*arrow*).

Table 1
Ulnar collateral ligament

Bundle	Location	Function	View
Anterior	From epicondyle to coronoid process	Major medial stabilizer	Coronal
Posterior	Cubital tunnel floor	Secondary stabilizer	Axial
Transverse	Between anterior and posterior bundles	No contribution to stability	—

ulnohumeral articulation, the medial collateral ligament, and the lateral collateral ligament. Secondary static constraints include the radial head, the common flexor and extensor origins, and the joint capsule. Dynamic stabilizers include the muscles that cross the elbow joint and produce compressive forces at the articulation. Of these, the anconeus, triceps, and brachialis are the most important. An elbow with all 3 of its primary constraints intact will be stable. When they are disrupted, the secondary stabilizers assume a more vital role.[8,9]

Elbow instability can be classified according to its longevity and course (acute, chronic, or recurrent); the articulations involved; the direction of displacement (valgus, varus, anterior, posterolateral, or rotatory); and the degree of displacement (subluxation or dislocation). It also may be categorized as simple (with no associated fracture) or complex (with an associated fracture).[8,9]

Valgus Instability

When valgus forces generated across a flexed elbow exceed the load-to-failure strength of the UCL, damage to the ligament occurs and valgus instability may develop. Such instability can occur from a single traumatic event, such as falling onto an outstretched arm, or chronically as a result of repetitive microtrauma, as seen in repetitive overhead throwers, like baseball pitchers, during the late cocking and acceleration phases of throwing.[8,9]

Gross inspection of ulnar collateral ligamentous anatomy is a challenge, even during surgery. Tenderness with palpation of the UCL, particularly with chronic instability, is not uniformly present. With recent tears, edema and ecchymosis may be noted. The mainstays of clinical evaluation are valgus stress tests. However, although a variety of maneuvers have been described, their accuracy varies widely even in the hands of experienced examiners.[8]

Given how difficult it is to evaluate UCL integrity, both in the clinic and during surgery, the importance of MR imaging cannot be understated. MR imaging findings vary with the severity of the injury (**Figs. 7** and **8**, **Table 4**). Alterations in morphology and signal intensity on T1-weighted and T2-weighted imaging indicate ligamentous disease. In the absence of discontinuity of the ligament, a sprain may be diagnosed. Clearing distinguishing ligament sprains from partial or even intrasubstance tears remains difficult on nonarthrographic MR imaging.[9]

Although the UCL may avulse either proximally or distally, midsubstance disruptions account for most traumatic injuries.[8] In adults, if avulsion-type injuries occur, they do so at the ulnar attachment onto the sublime tubercle.[9]

Insufficiency of the UCL complex has been associated with other abnormalities. Over time,

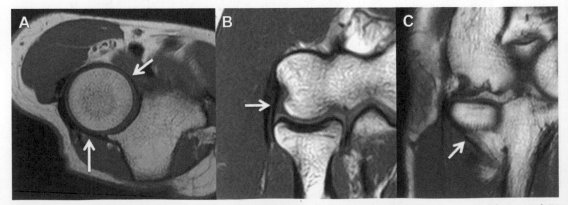

Fig. 4. Normal RCL complex. (*A*) Axial T1-weighted image of the annular ligament (*arrows*). (*B*) Coronal T1-weighted image of the RCL (*arrow*). (*C*) Coronal T1-weighted image of the LUCL (*arrow*).

Table 2
Radial collateral ligament

Ligament	Location	Function	View
Annular	Around radial head	Primary stabilizer PRUJ	Axial Sagittal[3]
Radial	From epicondyle to annular ligament	Annular ligament stabilizer[3]	Coronal
Lateral ulnar	From epicondyle to supinator crest	Major posterolateral stabilizer	Coronal Sagittal

secondary stabilizers are activated and the articular geometry changes, leading to degenerative changes within the radiocapitellar articulation, where osteochondral lesions may develop. In addition, medial joint instability can cause injuries of the ulnar nerve.

Posterolateral Rotatory Instability

Posterolateral rotatory instability (PLRI) is the most common pattern of elbow instability, and the most frequent form causing recurrent instability.[8] Factors that may contribute to PRLI include a history of previous trauma, chronic resistant lateral epicondylitis, and prior lateral elbow surgery, with posttraumatic laxity, disruption, or avulsion of the LUCL considered the main contributing factor.[8,10]

Since first described by O'Driscoll and colleagues in 1991,[11] the understanding of PLRI pathoanatomy has increased steadily over the last 2 decades. The typical mechanism of injury

Table 3
Muscles compartments of the elbow

Compartment	Muscles
Lateral	Extensor carpi radialis longus, extensor carpi radialis brevis, extensor digitorum communis, extensor carpi ulnaris, extensor digiti minimi, anconeus,[4] supinator
Medial	Pronator teres, flexor carpi radialis, palmaris longus, flexor carpi ulnaris, flexor digitorum superficialis, flexor digitorum profundus, flexor pollicis longus, brachioradialis
Anterior	Brachialis, biceps
Posterior	Triceps

Adapted from Walz DM, Newman JS, Konin GP, et al. Epicondylitis: pathogenesis, imaging, and treatment. Radiographics 2010;30:169, 177.

is falling onto an outstretched hand with the shoulder abducted, resulting in axial compression. External rotation and valgus forces are applied to the elbow as the body rotates internally on the hand and approaches the ground. Disruption of the supporting structures occurs in a circular fashion, which is referred to as the "circle of Horii" (Fig. 9). A staging system (Table 5) described by O'Driscoll may influence the collection of a patient's history, clinical examination, and options for treatment.[8–10]

Patients with PLRI may have pain and discomfort in the elbow as well as sensations of locking, clicking, snapping, or slipping, typically noted at 40 of flexion as the arm goes into extension within the arc of motion. In asymptomatic patients, nonoperative measures can include avoidance of instability-causing activities, elbow bracing to limit supination and valgus loading, application of a sugar tong cast, pain control, or physical therapy. If symptoms or instability persist, operative intervention is indicated.[10]

In clinical settings, clear imaging of the elbow is generally difficult. When the level of suspicion is high and radiograph results are normal, MR imaging should be performed. Although only a few studies have been done to identify MR imaging findings related to PLRI, in the presence of significant disease, damage of the lateral ligamentous complex may be clearly evident (Fig. 10).[3,8]

The most significant complications are recurrence and arthrosis; others include infection, bony bridge fracture, cutaneous nerve injury, and arthrofibrosis that results in a flexion contracture.[10]

EPICONDYLITIS

Lateral and medial epicondylitis are common causes of pain and functional impairment and typically result from specific occupational or sports-related activities. Epicondylitis most commonly occurs in either the fourth or the fifth decade of life, without predilection with regards to gender. It is widely thought to originate from repetitive overuse that results in microtears and progressive

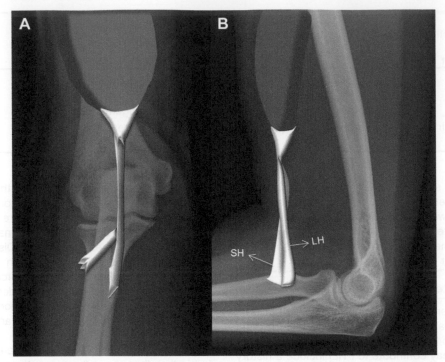

Fig. 5. DBT appears as a single unit (*A*), although it should be thought of as having 2 heads (*B*). As the tendon approaches the radial tuberosity, it gradually externally rotates 90 , causing the short head (SH, *arrow*) to insert distal to the long head (LH, *arrow*). The SH plays a greater role in flexion of the elbow; meanwhile, the LH acts as a powerful supinator.

degeneration secondary to an inadequate reparative response. These microtears and progressive degeneration, in turn, lead to tendinosis and partial tearing that ultimately may progress to a full-thickness tendon tear. Histologically, there is fibrillar degeneration of collagen, angiofibroblastic proliferation, tissue necrosis with myxoid and

hyaline degeneration, and fibrosis, all in the absence of inflammatory cells.[4]

Medial epicondylitis, or tennis elbow, typically occurs in throwing athletes, tennis players, golfers, and bowlers, as well as in workers whose occupations result in similar repetitive motions. In such cases, the pronator teres and flexor carpi radialis

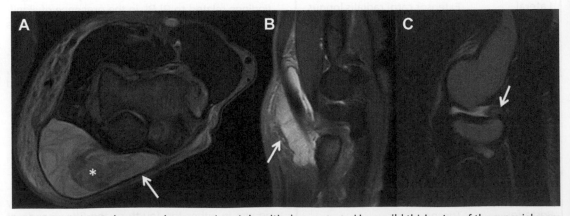

Fig. 6. (*A*) Axial STIR shows an olecranon chronic bursitis demonstrated by a mild thickening of the synovial membrane (*arrow*) and heterogeneous signal (*asterisk*). (*B*) Sagittal STIR shows a bicipitoradial acute bursitis visible as a fluid collection with thin walls (*arrow*). (*C*) Sagittal T2-weighted image shows enlarged posterolateral plicae with high signal intensity (*arrow*).

Box 2
Elbow instability: teaching points

1. The most important static soft tissue constraints are the LUCL and the anterior bundle of the UCL.

2. Caution should be exercised when making the diagnosis of partial UCL detachment: remember the striated appearance of the ligament.

3. UCL midsubstance disruptions account for most traumatic injuries.

4. Conventional MR imaging shows sensitivity, specificity, and accuracy that approach 100% for full-thickness UCL tears.

5. The anterior bundle of the UCL is often intact even when the radial head and coronoid process are both fractured.

6. Posttraumatic laxity, disruption, or avulsion of the LUCL is considered to be the main contributing factor in PLRI.

7. The most common injury to the LUCL is soft tissue avulsion at the proximal humeral attachment, often with concomitant injury to the common origin of the RCL.

8. Elbow dislocation is most commonly associated with a torn capsule, but the capsule may be intact if the coronoid process is fractured.

9. An abnormal posterolateral plicae usually reflects incompetence of the UCL.

are most commonly injured, followed by the palmaris longus. Lateral epicondylitis, or tennis elbow (**Fig. 11**), generally occurs in individuals performing any activity that involves repeated supination and pronation of the forearm with the elbow in extension. Its incidence is 7 to 10 times that of medial epicondylitis, and the essential lesion involves the extensor carpi radialis brevis (ECRB).[4,8]

The ECRB has a complex origin, receiving contributions from the common extensor tendon, lateral collateral ligament, annular ligament, overlying fascia, and intramuscular septum. These contributions are intertwined and not always separable; consequently, capsular injury as well as thickening and tearing of the ligament has been identified in severe cases.[4]

The pathologic features of medial and lateral epicondylitis are similar (**Table 6**), and imaging is not always essential during the initial evaluation unless the clinical picture is unclear or the condition refractory to conservative treatment. In these situations, MR imaging should be performed to verify the diagnosis, quantify the degree of tendon injury, identify associated abnormalities that may explain the lack of response to conservative therapy, and aid in preoperative planning.[4]

OSTEOCHONDRAL INJURIES

Although confusion remains between the terms osteochondral injury and osteochondritis dissecans, it is really the cause of the process that is in question.[8] An osteochondral injury involves separation of a segment of articular cartilage along with its underlying bone and is a general term used to characterize the pathologic abnormality with no consideration of underlying cause.[8] The basic types of osteochondral injury that occur in the elbow are classified by acuity as well as by the clinical history and age of the patient at symptom onset. The imaging approach to osteochondral

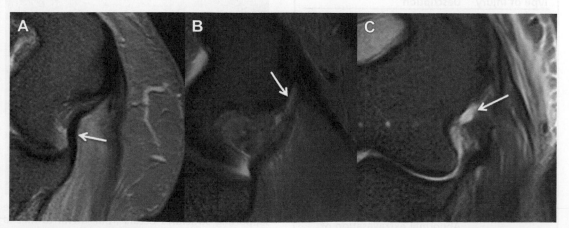

Fig. 7. Coronal STIR images of the anterior bundle of the UCL. (*A*) Normal ligament (*arrow*). (*B*) Ligament with a partial undersurface tear (*arrow*). (*C*) Ligament with a complete proximal tear (*arrow*, see **Table 4**).

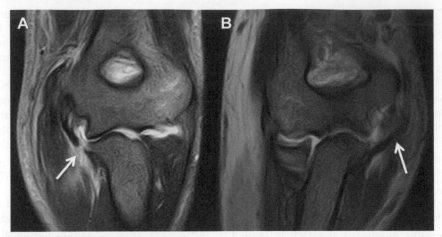

Fig. 8. Coronal STIR images profile a complete rupture of the UCL (*arrow*) near the sublime tubercle (*A, B*) at the proximal attachment (*arrow*) associated with extravasation of joint fluid.

injuries, regardless of cause, should be the same, beginning with radiographs. However, 2 crucial points about radiographs should be made. First, lesions that are observable on radiographs do not have a good prognosis with conservative management, and delayed surgery may worsen the prognosis.[8] Second, negative radiographs do not rule out an osteochondral lesion; consequently, MR imaging is needed to confirm or exclude any clinically suspected diagnosis.

Posttraumatic Fractures

Impaction injuries can involve the posterior capitellum, at the junction of the capitellum and distal radius, and are often associated with fractures or contusions involving the anterior aspect of the

radial head and coronoid process. Accompanying injuries of the LUCL have been reported in up to 82% of patients. These injuries can be distinguished from capitellar pseudodefects by the presence of marrow edema as well as by articular and subchondral abnormalities (see **Box 1**; **Fig. 12**). MR imaging is also the modality of choice for the detection of radiographically occult fractures that often are suspected on the basis of persistent pain or joint effusion.

Table 4	
MR imaging findings of valgus instability	
Type of Injury	**Description**
Sprain	Absence of discontinuity Alterations in morphology: thinning or thickening High signal intensity on T1-weighted or T2-weighted images
Partial tear	Focal areas of discontinuity with residual intact fibers Edema
Complete tear	Discontinuity Alterations in morphology: Thickening Alteration in signal intensity: High signal in fluid sensitive sequences Abnormal extravasation of joint fluid

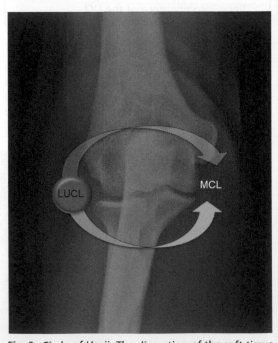

Fig. 9. Circle of Horii. The disruption of the soft tissue supporting structures occurs from lateral to medial with increasing severity (see **Table 5**). MCL, medial collateral ligament.

Table 5		
Posterolateral rotatory instability staging system		
Stage	Description	Presentation
I	LUCL disruption	Posterolateral subluxation
II	Disruption of remaining RCL complex and joint capsule	Perched incomplete dislocation
III A	UCL disruption with intact anterior bundle	Posterior dislocation
III B	Disruption of the UCL	Valgus, varus, and rotatory instability are present
III C	Not originally described Flexor-extensor muscular origins stripped off the distal humerus	Severe instability

Osteocondritis Dissecans

This entity has remained at the center of considerable discussion and debate, principally as a result of controversy over its cause, difficulty in its treatment, and its poor long-term prognosis. In addition, its name is somewhat inaccurate in that it implies inflammation, despite the fact that no inflammatory cells have ever been identified on histologic sections. Although the exact mechanism of injury is unclear, osteocondritis dissecans (OCD) is thought to result from repetitive microtrauma to a poorly vascularized capitellar chondroepiphysis, which then may lead to osteonecrosis.

When it occurs in the elbow, OCD refers primarily to lesions involving the anterior aspect of the capitellum, although lesions of the trochlea, radial head, olecranon, and olecranon fossa have been described. OCD occurs in immature athletes and is rarely found in adults. It primarily affects young men between 12 and 15 years of age, at a time when the capitellar epiphysis is almost completely ossified, usually affecting the dominant arm. In most cases, there is a history of overuse of the involved upper extremity.

Pain is the primary symptom at presentation and the onset is generally insidious. The typical course is one of progressive worsening, with pain in most patients tending to be activity-related and relieved by rest. If crepitus to palpation accompanies clicking, popping, or locking, the clinician should be highly suspicious of articular cartilage fragmentation and intra-articular body formation.

Nelson and colleagues[12] described an MR imaging classification system (**Table 7**), but it overlooks several features that radiologists need to assess (**Table 8**), such as fragment size, location, stability, and viability,[13] because this information could ultimately predict which lesions are likely to heal with nonoperative treatment (generally is reserved for early lesions without mechanical symptoms). When it is safe for the patient to return to sporting activities should be determined by symptoms and not by imaging studies, because the latter can remain abnormal for years.[8] Surgical intervention is typical in those athletes with mechanical symptoms or intra-articular bodies who have failed at least 6 months of nonoperative treatment. Predictors of a poor long-term outcome include a large fragment, an unstable lesion on presentation, increasing symptom severity over time, and the development of osteoarthritis.

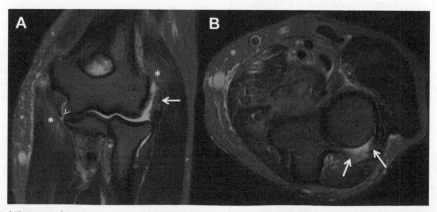

Fig. 10. PLRI. (*A*) Coronal STIR shows a full-thickness tear of the MCL anterior bundle (*arrow*), distal avulsion of the RCL (*arrowhead*), and muscle edema (*asterisks*). (*B*) Axial STIR shows a disruption of the annular ligament (*arrows*).

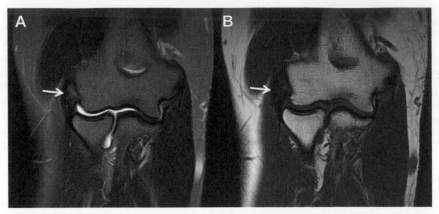

Fig. 11. Lateral epicondylitis. Coronal STIR (*A*) and T1-weighted (*B*) images demonstrating tendon thickening and tendinosis (*arrows*).

Panner Disease

Panner disease is a benign and self-limited condition of the entire capitellum (**Fig. 13**) that presents in childhood, primarily affecting male athletes under 10 years old before ossification of the capitellum is complete. Fragmentation, fissuring, and sclerosis can be observed; however, the articular surface remains intact and there is no articular body formation. Of note is that debate exists as to whether Panner disease and OCD may represent different stages of altered enchondral ossification.

INTRA-ARTICULAR BODIES

The elbow is the second most common site for intra-articular bodies,[8] because any process that leads to damage of the articular surface may result

in the formation of cartilaginous or osteocartilaginous bodies that may remain in situ. These bodies can be either partially or completely detached and, when free, can migrate, often collecting in synovial recesses (**Fig. 14**). Because they can grow as a result of the repetitive deposition of layers of fibrous and cartilaginous tissue, they should be removed, both to alleviate symptoms and to prevent further articular damage.

The accuracy of MR arthrography (92%) in the detection of osseous and cartilaginous bodies has proven to be significantly greater than that of standard MR imaging (57%–92%).[8]

DISTAL BICEPS TENDON

Evaluation of the DBT can be challenging. It also is sometimes difficult to differentiate high-grade partial tears from complete tears. Assessment of the distal tendon can be improved using the FABS position.[14]

Tears of the DBT occur distally within 1 to 2 cm of its insertion, where a hypovascular zone has been described within the tendon. The relative lack of vascularity can impede healing, potentially converting partial tears and fiber degeneration from repetitive trauma into complete tears. Conditions that result in relative tissue hypoxia, like smoking, have been shown to increase the risk of tendon ruptures. Systemic processes also may play a part (**Box 3**). Recurrent traction forces on the bicipital tuberosity can result in compensatory osseous hypertrophy and enthesophyte formation, which in turn increase the likelihood of mechanical impingement. Distension of the bicipitoradial or interosseous bursa (see **Fig. 6**) can also cause mass effect, further narrowing the radioulnar interval.

Most distal biceps tears are observed in men between the ages of 40 and 60. However, the

Table 6 Epicondylitis—MR imaging findings	
Type of Injury	**Description**
Tendinosis	Intermediate signal intensity in T1-weighted and T2-weighted images within the substance of the tendon with or without tendon thickening
Partial tear	Focal area of high signal intensity on fluid-sensitive sequences extending partway across the tendon with diffuse tendon thinning
Complete tear	Fluid signal intensity gap across the substance of the tendon or between the proximal tendon and its attachment

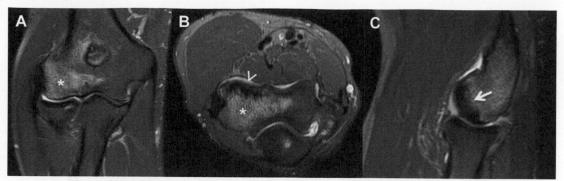

Fig. 12. STIR images in coronal (*A*), axial (*B*), and sagittal (*C*) planes reveal posttraumatic osteochondritis located in the anterior and inferior capitellum, with bone marrow edema (*asterisks*), subchondral sclerosis (*arrow*), and cartilage irregularity (*arrowhead*).

number of complete tears is increasing, likely reflecting increasing levels of activity in older men. DBT ruptures are classified as partial or complete. Partial ruptures currently have no classification system, whereas complete ruptures are subdivided into acute and chronic lesions, with acute ruptures presenting within 4 weeks of the injury and chronic injuries occurring after 4 weeks. Chronic injuries are further classified based on the integrity of the LF.

Complete tears (**Fig. 15**) usually occur as the result of a single traumatic event, characterized by a sudden eccentric load applied to a flexed elbow or forceful hyperextension against resistance. Clinically, patients feel a sudden "pop"

and sharp pain in the antecubital fossa, with weakness of elbow flexion and supination. If the biceps tendon is avulsed and the LF is torn, the tendon end retracts into the upper arm, producing a palpable defect, which makes the diagnosis relatively straightforward on clinical examination. However, if the LF remains intact, there may only be minimal retraction of the tendon, making the diagnosis more difficult.

MR imaging has been shown to be extremely sensitive (100%) in diagnosing complete tears, but less sensitive (59%) with partial tears.[15] Partial tears are uncommon, but also presumably underreported. Tears are uniformly located on the radial side of the tendon as it travels over the tuberosity. On MR imaging, the DBT may demonstrate increased intratendinous signal and can be either thickened or thinned, depending on the tear's severity (**Fig. 16**).

Table 7
OCD—MR imaging classification system

Grade	Description	Stability
0	Normal cartilage	—
I	Intact cartilage with signal change	Stable
II	High signal breach of overlying cartilage	Stable
III	Thin high signal rim of fluid extending about the OC fragment	Unstable
IV	Mixed or low signal intra-articular body	Fragment in situ or free

Adapted from Nelson DW, DiPaola J, Colville M. Osteochondritis dissecans of the talus and knee: prospective comparison of MR and arthroscopic classifications. J Comput Assist Tomogr 1990;14(5):804–8; with permission.

Table 8
OCD—MR imaging features associated with poor outcomes

Feature	Description
Fragment size	>1 cm
Location	Posteroinferior lateral trochlea (usually larger in size)
Unstable fragment	Peripheral rim of high signal intensity, underlying cyst, osteochondral fracture line, subchondral plate defect, fluid-filled osteochondral defect
Nonviable fragment	No gadolinium enhancement (intravenous injection)

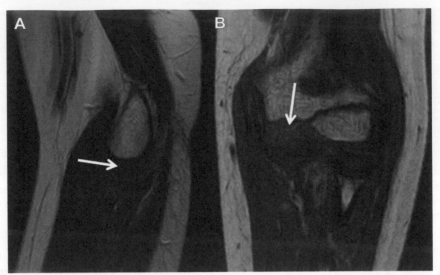

Fig. 13. Panner disease. Sagittal T2-weighted (A) and coronal T1-weighted (B) images show low signal intensity throughout the entire capitellar ossification center (arrows).

TRICEPS TENDON

Triceps tendon ruptures are the least common of all tendon injuries. There is a male predominance of 2:1 and a mean age at presentation of 36 years.[6,8] As with biceps, the systemic processes may play a role in triceps tendinopathy (see **Box 3; Fig. 17**).

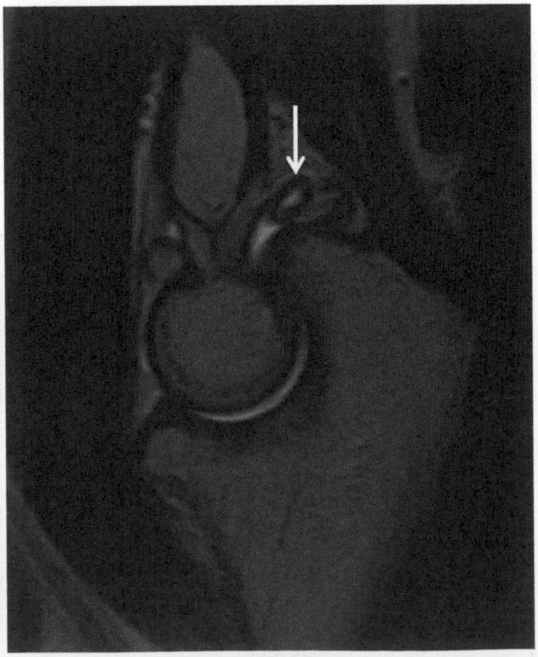

The most common mechanism of injury is falling onto an outstretched hand, during which a deceleration load is applied to the triceps while it is actively contracting. Motor vehicle accidents and weight-lifting, as well as direct blows to the triceps tendon and chronic lesions, have also been described (see **Fig. 17**).[6]

Distal triceps tendon tears are nearly always avulsions at the tendon-bone interface and have generally been characterized as complete or incomplete. Complete tears are reported more commonly. MR imaging most frequently reveals complete avulsion and retraction of the posterior component of the tendon (the combined attachment of the long and lateral heads) with the anterior component (medial head) remaining intact. Operative repair is recommended for tears greater than 50% on MR imaging that are associated with weakness (British MRC grade 3/5).[6]

Fig. 14. Intra-articular body. Sagittal T2-weighted image detects a heterogeneous round structure located within the olecranon fossa (arrow).

Box 3
Distal biceps tendon pathologic abnormality: risk factors
Ankylosing spondylitis
Rheumatoid arthritis
Acute rheumatic fever
Gout
Systemic lupus erythematosus
Chronic uremia
Hemodialysis
Hyperparathyroidism

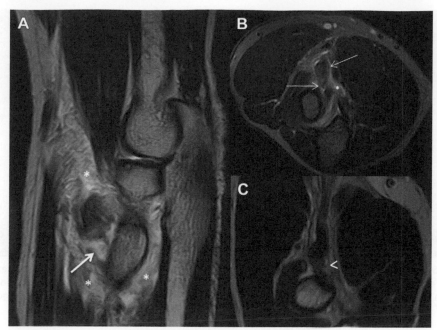

Fig. 15. Sagittal T2-weighted (*A*) and axial STIR (*B*) images demonstrate caliber changes in the DBT (*arrows*) associated with peritendinous edema (*asterisks*). (*C*) FABS shows a partial tear close to the insertion site (*arrowhead*).

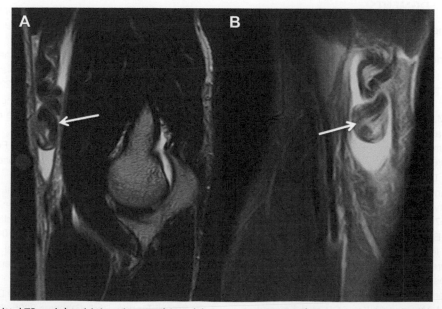

Fig. 16. Sagittal T2-weighted (*A*) and coronal STIR (*B*) demonstrates complete rupture of the distal biceps tendon, with the tendon end retracted into the upper arm (*arrow*) and surrounding hematoma. Biceps tendon retraction <8 cm typically correlates with an intact lacertus (LF), whereas retraction >8 cm indicates a torn LF.

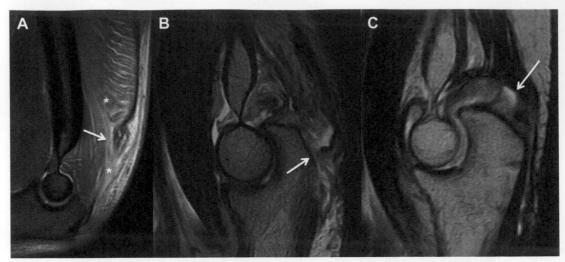

Fig. 17. (*A*) Sagittal PD-weighted fat-suppressed image shows an acute tear (*arrow*) with tendon retraction surrounded by edema (*asterisk*). (*B*) Sagittal T2-weighted image demonstrates a tear without retraction of the triceps tendon (*arrow*). (*C*) Sagittal T2-weighted image shows a chronic tendon tear related to gout (*arrow*). (*Courtesy of* [*A*] the MSK department, Italian Hospital, Buenos Aires.)

SUMMARY

The elbow is not only a complex anatomic region with a broad spectrum of common disorders but also an area that is difficult to assess, even by experienced examiners. For this reason, MR imaging plays an important role in both the diagnosis and the subsequent management of patients with elbow symptoms.

ACKNOWLEDGMENTS

The author gratefully thanks G. Rodriguez, S. Alvarez, F. Avila, and A. Rasumoff for their patience and support.

REFERENCES

1. Stein JM, Cook TS, Simonson S, et al. Normal and variant anatomy of the elbow on magnetic resonance imaging. Magn Reson Imaging Clin N Am 2011;19:609–19.

2. Husarik DB, Saupe N, Pfirrmann CW, et al. Ligaments and plicae of the elbow: normal MR imaging variability in 60 asymptomatic subjects. Radiology 2010;257:185–94.

3. Mak S, Beltran LS, Bencardino J, et al. MRI of the annular ligament of the elbow: review of anatomic considerations and pathologic findings in patients with posterolateral elbow instability. AJR Am J Roentgenol 2014;203:1272–9.

4. Walz DM, Newman JS, Konin GP, et al. Epicondylitis: pathogenesis, imaging, and treatment. Radiographics 2010;30:167–84.

5. Stevens K, Kwak A, Poplawski S. The biceps muscle from shoulder to elbow. Semin Musculoskelet Radiol 2012;16:296–315.

6. Stucken C, Ciccotti MG. Distal biceps and triceps injuries in athletes. Sports Med Arthrosc 2014;22(3): 153–63.

7. Husarik DB, Saupe N, Pfirrmann CW, et al. Elbow nerves: MR findings in 60 asymptomatic subjects—normal anatomy, variants, and pitfalls. Radiology 2009;252:148–56.

8. Chung CB, Steimbach L. MRI of the upper extremity: shoulder, elbow, wrist and hand. Philadelphia: Lippincott Williams & Wilkins; 2010.

9. Schaeffeler C, Waldt S, Woertler K. Traumatic instability of the elbow - anatomy, pathomechanisms and presentation on imaging. Eur Radiol 2013;23:2582–93.

10. Anakwenze OA, Kancherla VK, Iyengar J, et al. Posterolateral rotatory instability of the elbow. Am J Sports Med 2014;42:485–91.

11. O'Driscoll SW, Bell DF, Morrey BF. Posterolateral rotatory instability of the elbow. J Bone Joint Surg Am 1991;73(3):440–6.

12. Nelson DW, DiPaola J, Colville M, et al. Osteochondritis dissecans of the talus and knee: prospective comparison of MR and arthroscopic classifications. J Comput Assist Tomogr 1990;14(5):804–8.

13. Bancroft LW, Pettis C, Wasyliw C, et al. Osteochondral lesions of the elbow. Semin Musculoskelet Radiol 2013;17:446–54.

14. Chew ML, Giuffrè BM. Disorders of the Distal Biceps Brachii Tendon. RadioGraphics 2005;25:1227–37.

15. Schmidt CC, Jarrett CD, Brown DT. The Distal Biceps Tendon. JHS 2013;3:811–21.

Magnetic Resonance Arthrography of the Wrist and Elbow

Gary M. LiMarzi, MD[a,b], M. Cody O'Dell, MD[a,b],
Kurt Scherer, MD[a,b], Christopher Pettis, MD[a,b],
Christopher W. Wasyliw, MD[a,b], Laura W. Bancroft, MD[a,b],*

KEYWORDS

- MR arthrography • Scapholunate ligament tear • Ulnar collateral ligament tear
- Olecranon stress fracture • Osteochondritis dissecans

KEY POINTS

- Magnetic resonance (MR) arthrography is highly sensitive and specific for the diagnosis of scapholunate ligament tears.
- MR dictations should state if tears are partial-thickness or full-thickness, and if the tearing involves the dorsal, membranous, and/or volar components of the ligament.
- Partial-thickness tears of the anterior band of the ulnar collateral ligament in overhead-throwing athletes are well evaluated with MR arthrography.
- Repetitive valgus elbow stress and rapid elbow extension during the late stages of throwing may result in an olecranon stress fracture, with propagation from a structural weak point in the trochlear groove.
- Osteochondritis dissecans of the elbow is an osteochondral injury classically seen in adolescent or young adult athletes, especially baseball pitchers, due to repetitive valgus impaction injury of the radial head and developing ossification center of the capitellum.

MAGNETIC RESONANCE ARTHROGRAPHY OF THE WRIST

Wrist pain is a common, nonspecific patient complaint that may be secondary to a variety of underlying processes, both degenerative and traumatic. Wrist trauma can be divided into 2 categories: low impact and high impact. High-impact trauma can lead to displaced fractures, dislocations, and acute tears of the ligaments and tendons, whereas low-impact trauma can lead to more occult injuries.[1] Both mechanisms can result in injuries to the intrinsic and extrinsic carpal ligaments, as well as the triangular fibrocartilage complex (TFCC). Because the TFC is discussed in depth in the article by Cody et al, elsewhere in this issue, this article will not focus on its normal imaging appearance or pathology. Because clinical presentations can overlap significantly, magnetic resonance (MR) arthrography is essential in the diagnostic workup of such injuries. MR arthrography of the wrist is generally preferred over conventional MR imaging or computed tomography (CT) arthrography because of its high intrinsic contrast

The authors have nothing to disclose.
[a] Florida Hospital Diagnostic Radiology Residency Program, Department of Radiology, Florida Hospital, University of Central Florida College of Medicine, 601 East Rollins, Orlando, FL 32803, USA; [b] Department of Radiology, Florida Hospital, University of Central Florida College of Medicine, 6850 Lake Nona Boulevard, Orlando, FL 32827, USA
* Corresponding author.
E-mail address: Laura.bancroft.md@flhosp.org

Magn Reson Imaging Clin N Am 23 (2015) 441–455
http://dx.doi.org/10.1016/j.mric.2015.04.003
1064-9689/15/$ – see front matter © 2015 Elsevier Inc. All rights reserved.

mri.theclinics.com

resolution, as well as the ability to evaluate extra-articular soft tissue pathology. MR arthrography is indicated to evaluate TFCC, intrinsic and extrinsic carpal ligaments, and the distal radial ulnar joint (DRUJ).[2]

Technique

The use of intra-articular contrast agents provides an effective means of evaluating the TFCC and interosseous ligaments of the wrist. There is variability among institutions as to whether to perform single-compartment (most commonly radiocarpal), 2-compartment, or rarely 3-compartment (radiocarpal, DRUJ, and midcarpal) arthrography before MR arthrography. Injections are most commonly performed under fluoroscopic guidance, but some radiologists prefer sonographic guidance.[3] Radiocarpal injections are approached most commonly from a dorsal approach; however, some radiologists choose a lateral approach.[4] With the patient supine on the fluoroscopy table, the patient's wrist is placed in a flexed position and bolstered with a rolled towel. The radiocarpal joint is visualized in profile and the skin overlying the joint is marked at the level of the mid scaphoid. After prepping and draping the dorsum of the wrist, local anesthesia is administered with a 25-gauge, 1.5-inch anesthesia needle from a dorsal approach, and the needle is advanced into the radiocarpal joint. Connector tubing flushed with injectate from the syringe is connected to the needle after dripping contrast into the needle hub to displace any air. Although some radiologists inject only a small amount of iodinated contrast to confirm needle placement before injecting the dilute gadolinium mixture, it is also acceptable to combine the iodinate contrast and gadolinium together. While taking rapid cine images, an approximately 3-mL mixture of iodinated contrast and dilute gadolinium is injected into the radiocarpal joint, or until resistance is perceived (**Fig. 1**). The gadolinium-based contrast used in MR arthrography is usually diluted in normal saline and/or iodinated contrast to a concentration of 1:250, which optimizes the paramagnetic effects of gadolinium at 1.5-T field strengths. After removal of the needle, the wrist is then briefly exercised and conventional arthrographic images are obtained in the anteroposterior, lateral, and oblique images before MR arthrography. Some radiologists also prefer taking dedicated spot imaging of the scapholunate (SL) ligament with ulnar deviation or clenched fist stress maneuver. This arthrographic imaging is diagnostic, and is instrumental in cases of patients unable to complete the MR portion of the examination for a variety of reasons.

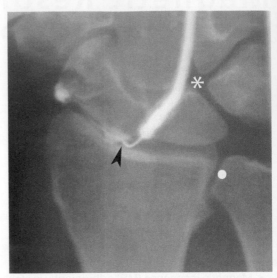

Fig. 1. Wrist arthrogram in a 70-year-old man before MR arthrography. Anteroposterior view of the wrist at the beginning of arthrogram demonstrates radiocarpal injection of 1:250 ratio of gadolinium to iodinated contrast through a 25-gauge needle (*arrowhead*) before MR arthrogram. Asterisk indicates site for midcarpal injection, and circle indicates site for distal radioulnar injection.

Midcarpal joint injections are most commonly performed from a dorsal approach into to the central portion of the 4-part junction of the lunate, triquetrum, hamate, and capitate. Distal radioulnar joint injection is performed from a dorsal approach, with the needle extending to the radial aspect of the ulnar head.

Contraindications

Besides the normal contraindications for MR imaging, the only absolute contraindication for arthrography is local infection of the skin or subcutaneous tissue.[5] One would not want to contaminate a joint by crossing a needle through infected tissues. Usually, patients who cannot undergo MR arthrography are able to tolerate imaging with CT arthrography. For example, patients with implantable cardiac pacemakers who, with some recent exceptions due to new MR imaging-safe pacemakers, cannot undergo MR arthrography, can be safely evaluated with CT.[5–8] A history of adverse contrast reactions with either iodinated or gadolinium-based agents is considered a relative contraindication and should be evaluated on a case-by-case basis.[5]

Complications

Arthrography is a generally well-tolerated procedure with few significant risks, and complications following arthrography are uncommon and usually in the form of pain. This can be due to overdistention of the joint space, irritation of surrounding nerves, or from intravasation of injected contrast into adjacent muscles.[5,7,8] Synovitis caused by the contrast also may be irritating and painful. Infection is an inherent risk to all percutaneous procedures, but is very rare.

Magnetic Resonance Acquisition

Wrist MR arthrography should be obtained on a 1.5-T or preferably a 3.0-T magnet in a dedicated wrist coil for optimal image quality, and thin-section imaging and small field of view should be used (**Table 1**).[9–13] Patients are optimally scanned in the prone position with the arm extended overhead and the wrist in neutral positioning near the isocenter of the magnet ("Superman" position).[13] If patients cannot tolerate this positioning, imaging is done with the wrist by the patient's side, with care to optimize fat suppression. MR arthrography includes axial, coronal, and sagittal imaging planes, and the coronal and sagittal sequences are prescribed relative to a plane intersecting the hook of the hamate and the palmar margin of the trapezium (**Fig. 2**). Most sequences are obtained with turbo spin echo (TSE) T1-weighting with fat suppression, to take advantage of the T1 properties of the injected gadolinium; T1-weighted images without fat suppression and T2-weighted images with fat suppression also are obtained. T2-weighted fat-suppressed and non–fat-suppressed T1-weighted images are useful in evaluating the marrow. T2-weighted images can detect noncommunicating tears of the intrinsic ligaments and TFCC on the opposite side of the injected joint, marrow edema, and noncommunicating periarticular fluid collections. Some centers

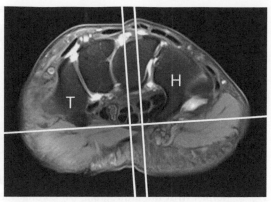

Fig. 2. Axial scout for prescription of coronal and sagittal views. A plane intersecting the hook of the hamate (H) and the palmar margin of the trapezium (T) serves as the reference plane for coronal acquisitions (*single line*). Sagittal images are prescribed from the axis perpendicular (*double lines*) to the coronal plane.

also prefer using gradient-echo sequences or 3-dimensional volumetric sequences. Although uncommonly used, some investigators use finger trap distraction with weights suspended from the fingers to accentuate the amount of contrast in the SL interval, widening of the space, and disruption of Gilula carpal arcs.[14,15]

NORMAL ANATOMY
Intrinsic Ligaments

The intrinsic and extrinsic interosseous ligaments of the wrist provide stability to the carpus. The SL ligament is the most commonly injured intrinsic carpal ligament and can predispose to carpal instability.[1,16–20] Patients with ligamentous injury typically present with dorsal wrist pain, crepitus with motion, weakness, and swelling. The SL ligament consists of the bandlike dorsal and volar components connected by the membranous portion composed of a proximal fibrocartilaginous membrane; the dorsal component is considered the primary SL stabilizer (**Fig. 3**).[16–20] The lunotriquetral (LT) ligament is similar in composition to the SL ligament; however, the volar rather than the dorsal component is considered the primary stabilizer of the LT ligament.[16–21] These ligaments provide a barrier between the radiocarpal and midcarpal spaces.[20] CT and MR arthrography have been shown to be more sensitive than standard MR for detecting abnormalities of these ligaments, and MR is superior to CT in detecting other causes of patient's symptoms, such as osteonecrosis, tendon and tendon sheath pathology, synovitis, fluid collections, and masses.[20]

Table 1
Sample wrist MR arthrogram protocol, using 1.5-T or 3.0-T magnet and dedicated wrist coil after radiocarpal injection of dilute gadolinium mixture

Plane	Sequence	FOV, cm	Slice Thickness, mm
Axial	TSE T1 FS	15	3
Coronal	TSE T1 FS	15	2
Sagittal	TSE T1 FS	15	3
Coronal	TSE T2 FS	15	2
Coronal	TSE T1	15	2

Abbreviations: FOV, field of view; FS, fat saturation; TSE, turbo spin echo.

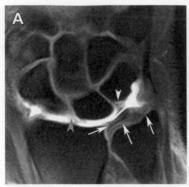
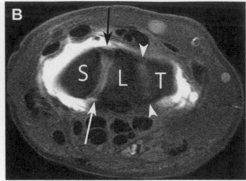

Fig. 3. Normal wrist MR arthrogram. (*A*) Coronal TSE fat-suppressed image after radiocarpal joint injection of dilute gadolinium mixture demonstrates normal appearance of the SL ligament (*gray arrowhead*), LT ligament (*white arrowhead*), and the TFC (*arrows*). (*B*) Axial image through the SL (*arrows*) and LT (*arrowheads*) ligaments show the thicker bandlike portions of the dorsal ligaments compared with the volar components. L, lunate; S, scaphoid; T, triquetrum.

Extrinsic Ligaments

The extrinsic ligaments of the wrist are shown to better advantage with MR arthrography due to joint distention. Dorsally, the extrinsic ligaments are the dorsal radiocarpal ligament (DRCL) and the dorsal intercarpal ligament (DICL) (**Fig. 4**).[13,22,23] These ligaments generally demonstrate homogeneously low signal intensity on MR imaging.[13,22,23] Volar extrinsic ligaments include the radioscaphocapitate ligament (RSCL), radiolunotriquetral ligament (RLTL, also known as the long radiolunate ligament), and the short radiolunate ligament. The RSCL is the most important volar extrinsic ligament, and the RSCL and RLTL can contain normal bands of higher signal on MR imaging/MR arthrography.[13,22,23] The radial collateral ligament (RCL) of the wrist arises as a focal condensation of the joint capsule, just deep to the extensor tendon sheath; it

originates from the radial styloid and inserts onto the scaphoid waist.[13,22] Carpal instability may occur when there is concomitant injury to the intrinsic and extrinsic interosseous ligaments.[1,22]

PATHOLOGY
Scapholunate Ligament

MR arthrography's ability to localize the precise location of the tear can help distinguish stable from potentially unstable injuries. Tears of the membranous portion of the SL ligament are usually degenerative and are not associated with carpal instability.[17] Complete SL ligament tears are identified on conventional and MR arthrography by contrast extending from the radiocarpal to the midcarpal joint space through a SL interval defect. In advanced cases, widening of the SL interval also can be seen.[17] Partial tears result in variable

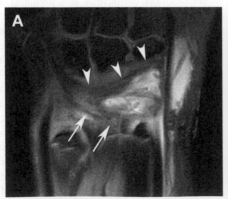
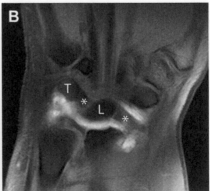

Fig. 4. Extrinsic ligaments. (*A*) Coronal image through the dorsal joint capsule of the wrist shows the normal dorsal radiocarpal (*arrows*) and dorsal intercarpal (*arrowheads*) ligaments. These intact ligaments are shown to better advantage with MR arthrography due to joint distention. (*B*) Coronal MR arthrogram through the volar wrist shows the volar radiolunotriquetral (RLT) ligament (*asterisks*). L, lunate; T, triquetrum.

intravasation of contrast through the torn fibers and outline the abnormal morphology of the tear. SL ligament injuries typically occur in the setting of axial overload or hyperextension with supination, often in the setting of a fall.[1] There also is increased association of SL ligament tears with intra-articular fractures. When isolated, SL ligament tears usually do not cause carpal malalignment (**Figs. 5** and **6**). Disruption of the secondary stabilizers of the scaphoid leads to rotation of the scaphoid with proximal subluxation, as well as dorsal extension of the lunate, resulting in dorsal intercalated segmental instability (DISI).[1,16,17,24]

Magnetic Resonance Arthrography Accuracy: Scapholunate Ligament

Although conventional MR imaging can detect partial and complete tears of the intrinsic carpal ligaments by the presence of focal thinning or discontinuity, MR arthrography is widely preferred due to improved sensitivity.[17] Arthrographic sensitivity for SL ligament tears has been shown to range widely. Scheck and colleagues[12] demonstrated 90% sensitivity/87% specificity with MR arthrography, compared with 52% sensitivity/34% specificity on conventional MR imaging. Lee and colleagues[8] also demonstrated superior accuracy of MR arthrography (85.0% sensitivity/96.4% specificity) when compared with conventional MR imaging (65% sensitivity/100% specificity) in the evaluation of SL ligament tears. Compared with arthroscopy, Magee and colleagues[25] reported that MR arthrography with 3 T yielded 100% sensitivity and specificity for the detection of SL ligament tears.

Dorsal Intercalated Segmental Instability

The 4 main categories of carpal instability include dissociative carpal instability, nondissociative

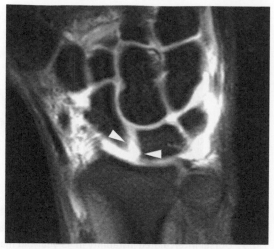

Fig. 6. Complete SL ligament rupture. Coronal MR arthrogram shows contrast filling the widened SL interval (*arrowheads*) due to complete rupture of the SL ligament and SL dissociation.

carpal instability, complex carpal instability, and adaptive carpal instability.[16,24] Although carpal instability may be suggested radiographically in cases of static instability, patients will invariably undergo MR imaging for evaluation of dynamic instability and treatment planning. DISI is one of the dissociative instabilities that occurs when there is disruption of the SL.[17] As on radiographs, MR will also show dorsal tilt of the lunate with a capito-lunate angle greater than 30, hyperflexion of the scaphoid, and incongruity of Gilula arcs in the presence of DISI deformity (**Fig. 7**). MR arthrography may be helpful to also assess tears or excessive stretching of the secondary stabilizers of the scaphoid, such as the volar distal scaphotrapezial, dorsal intercarpal and SL ligaments.[17]

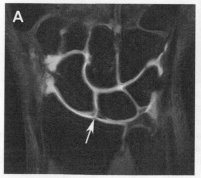
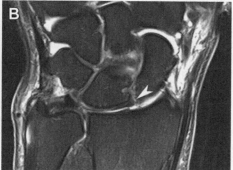

Fig. 5. SL ligament tears. (*A*) Coronal MR arthrogram in a 29-year-old man with wrist pain demonstrate full-thickness tear of the SL ligament (*arrow*), with opacification of the midcarpal joint space due to the communication from the tear. (*B*) Coronal TSE T2-weighted image from MR arthrogram in 70-year-old man with wrist pain shows irregular tearing of the volar aspect of the SL ligament (*arrowhead*).

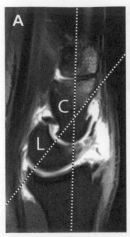
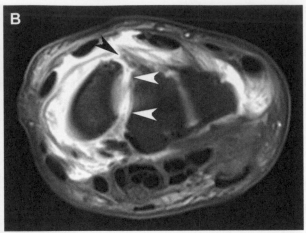

Fig. 7. Dorsal intercalated instability in 43-year-old man with traumatic SL and extrinsic dorsal ligament tears. (*A*) Sagittal MR arthrogram shows dorsal tilt of the lunate 'L' relative to the capitates 'C,' with increased lunate-capitate angle greater than 30 . (*B*) Axial MR arthrogram also shows rupture of the DRCL (*black arrowhead*) and full-thickness tears of the dorsal and membranous portions of the SL ligament (*white arrowheads*), accounting for contrast extension into the midcarpal joint.

Lunatotriquetral Ligament

Injuries to the LT ligament are much less common than those involving the SL ligament; LT ligament tears may be misdiagnosed clinically as TFCC pathology in patients presenting with ulnar-sided wrist pain.[1,17] As with SL ligament injury, isolated LT ligament tears are generally stable. Disruption of the secondary triquetral stabilizer, the radiolunotriquetral ligament, predisposes to volar intercalated segmental instability, in which there is palmar rotation of the lunate and scaphoid.[16,17,24]

Magnetic Resonance Arthrography Accuracy: Lunatotriquetral Ligament

Conventional MR imaging is unreliable in excluding pathology of the LT ligament due to inconsistent visualization in healthy patients. MR arthrography has been shown to have sensitivity for LT ligament tears of up to 56%, when considering both complete and partial tears (**Fig. 8**).[17] A series of 35 patients demonstrated a sensitivity and specificity of 100% for complete tears of the SL and LT ligaments with 3-T MR arthrography.[13] LT ligament tearing may be accompanied by tearing of the TFCC and lunate chondromalacia in the setting of ulnolunate impaction (see **Fig. 8**). Compared with arthroscopy, Magee and colleagues[25] reported that MR arthrography yielded 100% sensitivity and specificity for the detection of LT ligament tears.

Ulnocarpal Impaction Syndrome

Ulnocarpal impaction syndrome is caused by repetitive impaction injury between the ulnar

head, TFCC, and carpus, resulting in a spectrum of pathology. Ulnocarpal impaction is usually seen in the setting of positive ulnar variance, either congenital or posttraumatic, with distal radial malunion.[16,17,24] The TFC is thinner in patients with

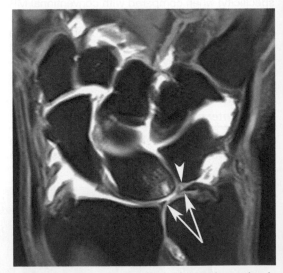

Fig. 8. LT ligament tear and ulnolunate impaction in 49-year-old man with chronic wrist pain. Coronal MR arthrogram shows a linear tear of the LT ligament (*arrowhead*) with extension of contrast into the midcarpal joint and Palmer 2E TFCC defect (*arrows*) with injected contrast and synovitis in the DRUJ. The subchondral cyst and enhancing marrow in the proximal, medial lunate, chondromalacia involving the abutting surfaces of the ulnar and lunate, and mild ulnar positive variance are classic findings of ulnolunate impaction.

positive ulnar variance and loading of the ulnar carpus is increased, both factors that may predispose to increased rates of TFCC pathology.[11,17,21] Increasing the ulnar variance by 2.5 mm will increase the ulnar load by 42%, more than twice the normal amount.[9] In rare cases, similar degenerative findings may be seen in the setting of a hypertrophic ulnar styloid with negative ulnar variance, referred to as ulnar styloid impaction syndrome (see **Fig. 8**).

MAGNETIC RESONANCE ARTHROGRAPHY OF THE ELBOW

In North America, MR arthrographic evaluation of the elbow is most commonly performed to investigate pain in throwing athletes and patients sustaining trauma from severe valgus stresses, posterorlateral rotator subluxation, and dislocation.[5] Typically, the pain is medial and occurs during the late-cocking phase of throwing, at the point of maximal valgus stress on the medial elbow stabilizers. Unsurprisingly, baseball pitchers, both amateur and professional, comprise a significant portion of patients undergoing arthrography in this part of the world.[5,26] Elsewhere, elbow arthrography is generally used to evaluate acute traumatic injury, namely posterolateral rotatory subluxation and severe valgus injuries.[5] Although less commonly performed than arthrography of the shoulder and knee, elbow arthrography is an important means of investigating intra-articular and ligamentous pathology. Direct arthroscopy is rarely performed as a first-line examination because of the excellent ability of MR and CT arthrography to demonstrate relevant pathology that can then guide arthroscopic evaluation or surgical intervention. Distention of the joint capsule with intra-articular contrast greatly improves visualization of articular and ligamentous structures, which would be overlooked on conventional imaging, increasing the sensitivity of the examination.[5] Contrast in the joint space helps separate closely related structures and provides improved image contrast. Detection of subtle pathology, including partial ligament tears and early osteochondral injury, also is improved.

MR arthrography is typically considered superior to CT arthrography because of improved soft tissue contrast resolution and the ability to obtain source images in multiple planes; however, CT possesses better spatial resolution and is the preferred modality for select patients.[26] Individuals with pacemakers, non-MR safe implantable devices, or who cannot tolerate gadolinium-based contrast agents are excellent candidates for CT arthrography.[5,26] Both modalities are considered far superior to conventional arthrography, which has been largely replaced in modern practice. The most common clinical indications for MR arthrography include detecting injuries to the capsule and supporting ligaments, the presence of intra-articular bodies, and focal osteochondral injury.[5,26]

Technique

The lateral approach into the radiocapitellar joint is the most commonly used approach for accessing the elbow joint. After palpating the radiocapitellar joint with patient pronating and supinating the forearm, the overlying skin is marked. The patient should preferably be positioned prone (in case of vasovagal reaction) or seated with the elbow flexed at 90 and in supination so that the thumb points toward the ceiling.[5] The radiocapitellar joint is visualized and marked under fluoroscopy. Using the general arthrographic principles described previously, local anesthetic is administered from a direct lateral approach with 25-gauge needle, and then the needle is advanced into the radiocapitellar joint. Intra-articular needle placement is confirmed when contrast can be seen flowing freely away from the needle (**Fig. 9**). The solution of diluted gadolinium is then injected for a total volume of 6 to 10 mL or until resistance is felt.

Occasionally, practitioners may elect to abandon the lateral approach in favor of a posteromedial approach.[27] This is usually done when there is clinical concern regarding the lateral ligament complex, because the lateral approach may lead to a small amount of contrast leaking through the percutaneous access site, which can lead to a false-positive diagnosis of lateral ligamentous pathology.[5,28] The patient is positioned supine with the shoulder abducted over the head and the elbow in pronation and approximately 30 of flexion. The medial epicondyle is identified and the skin entry site is marked approximately 1 cm lateral to the epicondyle on the posterior aspect of the arm, reducing the risk of injury to the ulnar nerve.[5] Once the patient is prepped and draped, the needle is directed anterolaterally toward the olecranon fossa. At this point, the examination proceeds in an identical fashion to that of a lateral approach.

Magnetic Resonance Acquisition

During the actual MR image acquisition, the patient may be positioned either prone with the elbow extended overhead, the "Superman" position, or supine with the elbow extended along the body (**Table 2**).[29] Images are obtained in axial, coronal, and sagittal planes. A plane intersecting the

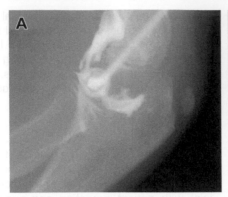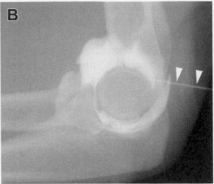

Fig. 9. Fluoroscopically guided elbow arthrography from standard lateral (*A*) and posterior (*B*) approaches in a 9-year-old boy and an 11-year-old girl, respectively. (*A*) After palpating the radiocapitellar joint, with the patient pronating and supinating the forearm, the overlying skin is marked for direct lateral approach into the radiocapitellar joint with 25-gauge needle. (*B*) The posterior approach (*arrowheads*) is an alternate route that will avoid misinterpretation of extravasated contrast about the lateral collateral ligament as pathology.

medial and lateral humeral epicondyles serves as the reference plane for coronal acquisitions, and sagittal images are prescribed from the axis perpendicular to the coronal plane (**Fig. 10**). MR arthrography uses T1-weighted sequences, which provide a higher signal-to-noise ratio than T2-weighted sequences and also require less time, therefore causing less motion artifact.[5,30] Fat-suppressed T1-weighted sequences are performed in the axial, coronal, and sagittal planes. Fat-suppressed T2-weighted images also are obtained, usually in the axial and coronal planes. By combining contrast-enhanced and fluid-sensitive sequences, the elbow can be evaluated for stress fractures/contusions and extra-articular pathology, such as nerve and muscle pathology, and tendon injuries (particularly enthesopathic changes of the common extensor and flexor tendon origins).[5] Some institutions also prefer using gradient-echo sequences or 3-dimensional volumetric sequences.

Normal Anatomy

The elbow is a synovial-lined, encapsulated joint composed of 3 distinct articulations: the radiocapitellar, ulnohumeral, and proximal radioulnar joints.[30] Of these, the biggest contributor to elbow stability is the ulnohumeral joint, responsible for 55% to 75% of joint restriction in extension and flexion, respectively.[29] The radiocapitellar joint, although playing a lessor role in joint stability, is responsible for transmitting 60% of the axial load from the forearm.[29] There is a normal, mild degree of lateral angulation of the humerus and ulna, referred to as the valgus carrying angle of the

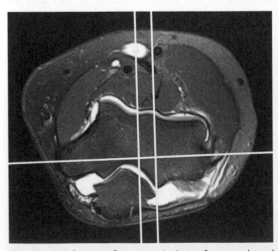

Fig. 10. Axial scout for prescription of coronal and sagittal views. A plane intersecting the medial and lateral humeral epicondyles serves as the reference plane for coronal acquisitions (*single line*). Sagittal images are prescribed from the axis perpendicular (*double lines*) to the coronal plane.

Table 2
Sample elbow MR arthrogram protocol using 1.5-T or 3.0-T magnet and dedicated elbow coil after injection of dilute gadolinium mixture

Plane	Sequence	FOV, cm	Slice Thickness, mm
Coronal	TSE T1 FS	15	2.5
Sagittal	TSE T1 FS	15	2.5
Axial	TSE T1 FS	15	2.5
Coronal	TSE T2 FS	15	2.5
Coronal	TSE T1	15	2.5

Abbreviations: FOV, field of view; FS, fat saturation; TSE, turbo spin echo.

elbow. This is usually between 10 and 20 and predisposes the elbow to valgus instability, whereas varus instability remains uncommon.[29]

Ligamentous supporting structures of the elbow arise as focal condensations of the joint capsule and are divided into medial and lateral complexes.[29,30] These provide stability under valgus and varus stresses, respectively. The medial complex consists of the anterior and posterior bundles of the ulnar collateral ligament (UCL, also known as the medial collateral ligament) as well as the transverse ligament (**Fig. 11A**). The lateral complex includes the RCL, the lateral UCL (LUCL), and the annular ligament (see **Fig. 11B**). The most important component of the medial ligament complex is the anterior bundle of the UCL, which provides the most resistance against valgus forces.[29,31] Both bundles of the UCL originate from the inferior aspect of the medial epicondyle; the anterior bundle inserts on the sublime tubercle of the ulna and the posterior bundle forms the floor of the cubital tunnel.[26,29] The posterior bundle inserts on the trochlear notch and helps resist internal rotation. The transverse ligament spans between the anterior and posterior bundles of the UCL and is poorly visualized with MR.[29] Superficially, the UCL is in close relationship to the flexor muscle group. On MR imaging, the UCL has a striated appearance in more than 90% of healthy volunteers, which should not be confused with injury.

The annular ligament serves an important role as a stabilizer of the proximal radioulnar joint and is more clinically relevant in pediatric patients than adults.[29] It inserts twice on the lesser sigmoid notch of the ulna after enveloping the radial head. The LUCL provides most of the support to the lateral elbow ligaments and is a key restraint against posterolateral rotatory instability.[29,30] It originates from the lateral epicondyle and courses posterior to the radial head before inserting on the supinator crest of the ulna. In this way, the LUCL prevents the ulna from rotating about its long axis away from the trochlea.[29] On conventional MR imaging, the LUCL is incompletely visualized in up to 23% of healthy volunteers.[29] Although the RCL also originates from the lateral epicondyle, this fan-shaped ligament runs longitudinally and blends distally with the annular ligament.

PATHOLOGY

The most common indication for MR arthrography of the elbow is medial joint pain, especially if occurring during overhand throwing. It is important to carefully assess all supporting structures, which should be easily visualized due to capsular distention by intra-articular contrast. Additionally, extra-articular etiologies for elbow pain should be evaluated as with any nonarthrographic study.

Ulnar Collateral Ligament Tear

Because the anterior bundle of the UCL is the most important stabilizer against valgus stress, it is no surprise that this ligament is most frequently injured in pitchers as a result of the high stresses placed on the joint during the late-cocking phase of throwing.[5,26,28,29] The UCL should be easily visualized on MR arthrography and is normally homogeneously hypointense along its superficial aspect proximally. The deep margin can be more heterogeneous in signal, which should not be confused with injury.[5,29]

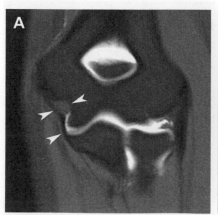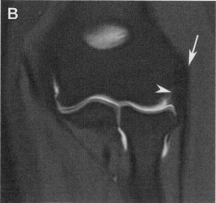

Fig. 11. Normal MR imaging arthrogram of the elbow in a 17 year-old girl with elbow pain. (*A*) Coronal image shows the normal fan-shaped configuration of the anterior bundle of the UCL (*arrowheads*), with normally increased signal intensity in the proximal ligament. (*B*) Coronal image show the normal RCL proper (*arrowhead*) deep to the intact common extensor tendon origin (*arrow*). MR arthrography adds value over conventional MR when there is the suspicion of partial-thickness tearing of the collateral ligaments in high-level athletes.

When the heterogeneity of the proximal UCL extends to involve the superficial aspect of the ligament, a partial-thickness tear should be suspected. Partial tears also can appear as a focal tear in the proximal UCL with its apex directed toward the superficial surface (**Fig. 12**).[5,26] Visualization of these partial tears is improved with arthrography, as contrast can be seen filling the tear and extending into the ligament (**Fig. 13**). These tears are of uncertain clinical significance, and athletes often continue to throw without surgical repair.[5,29]

The characteristic appearance of a partial tear of the distal UCL is referred to as the "T sign," due to contrast entering the defect and extending a short distance distally between the UCL and the proximal ulna (see **Fig. 12**). The anterior bundle normally inserts approximately 3 mm distal to the proximal margin of the sublime tubercle, so if there is contrast extending more than 3 mm distally, a partial tear should be suspected.[5,31] Whether or not these tears require surgical repair largely depends on the percentage of ligament involved and the degree to which contrast extends distal to the sublime tubercle. Schwartz and colleagues[32] demonstrated 86% sensitivity/100% specificity for detection of partial-thickness tears on arthrography.

Traumatic injury to the UCL also can be assessed with MR arthrography, although the abnormalities associated with acute trauma follow a less-reproducible pattern than those secondary to recurrent valgus stresses.[5] In cases of acute trauma, there are frequently associated injuries to the surrounding structures, including capsular disruption, fractures of the coronoid process of the ulna, articular cartilage delamination, and contusion.[5] The best indicator of traumatic disruption of the UCL is contrast extending medial to the joint line; the location of tear (ie, proximal or distal) is less important in the setting of trauma and these tears infrequently require reconstruction.

ULNAR COLLATERAL LIGAMENT RECONSTRUCTION

Reconstruction of the UCL is commonly performed in patients with medial elbow instability secondary to complete tears. In high-performing athletes, the tendency to return to a normal level of activity soon after surgery can lead to postoperative pathology.[33] In certain cases, evaluation with MR arthrography can be useful to evaluate the reconstruction as well as the adjacent elbow stabilizers. Due to the variable appearance of the reconstructed UCL in terms of thickness and signal characteristics, the best indicator of pathology is opacification of the fibers of the graft by intra-articular contrast (**Fig. 14**).[33] The reconstructed ligament is expected to be thickened and heterogeneous compared with the native ligament, and is anchored into the sublime tubercle more distal than the native ligament, allowing a small amount of contrast to extend into the recess normally. However, extravasation of medial joint fluid into the reconstructed ligament would be considered a tear.

Radial Collateral Ligament Complex

The radial collateral ligament complex is composed of the radial collateral ligament (RCL) proper, the lateral ulnar collateral ligament (LUCL), and the annular ligament.[34] The LUCL is

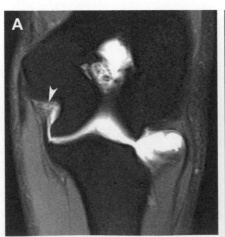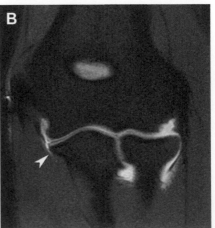

Fig. 12. Partial-thickness tear of the UCL. (*A*) Injected contrast extends into the deep proximal fibers (*arrowhead*) of the anterior band of the UCL in a 44-year-old who previously worked as a stuntman. (*B*) A 17-year-old baseball player producing the "T sign." Coronal MR arthrogram shows contrast dissecting proximally and distally along the undersurface of the UCL producing the "T sign" of a partial UCL tear (*white arrowhead*).

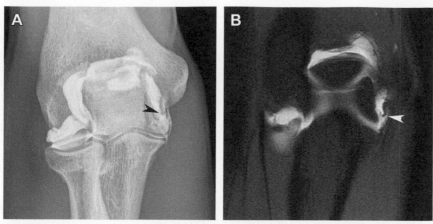

Fig. 13. Partial-thickness tear of the UCL. Fluoroscopic (*A*) and coronal MR arthrogram (*B*) both demonstrating contrast extending past the expected location of the UCL (*black arrowhead*). The MR arthrogram shows the partial tear with retraction of some of the torn fibers (*white arrowhead*).

the most frequently injured lateral ligament in the setting of traumatic subluxation or dislocation of the elbow.[5] The incidence of traumatic elbow dislocation is 5 to 6 per 100,000, surpassed only by dislocations of the shoulder.[29] The course of the LUCL along the inferior aspect of the proximal radius predisposes it to damage from translational forces. The normal LUCL should be taut and homogeneously low signal on MR arthrography; the presence of focal ligamentous thickening or laxity should raise suspicion for a tear. Complete tears can be seen as focal disruption with extravasation of contrast through the defect in the LUCL.[5] The RCL is located anterior to the LUCL and is also

susceptible to injury in the setting of trauma (**Fig. 15**).[5] Detection of any abnormality involving the RCL or LUCL should prompt close scrutiny of the remaining lateral ligament. Posterolateral elbow instability can occur in the setting of chronic recurrent injury to the LUCL, as the ability of the ligament to resist rotational forces is diminished over time.

Laxity of the LUCL near its ulnar insertion allows rotation and possible subluxation of the ulnohumeral joint with eventual secondary dislocation of the radiohumeral joint.[5] Importantly, the annular ligament is not disrupted and the proximal radioulnar joint remains intact.

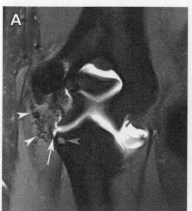
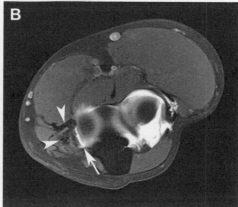

Fig. 14. Intact UCL reconstruction in a 27-year-old professional baseball pitcher. Coronal (*A*) and axial (*B*) images from MR arthrogram shows the normal postoperative appearance of an intact UCL ligament repair. The reconstructed ligament is expected to be thickened and heterogeneous (*white arrowheads*) compared with the native ligament, and is anchored into the sublime tubercle (*gray arrowhead*) more distal than the native ligament, allowing a small amount of contrast (*arrow*) to extend into the recess. (*B*) Axial image shows no extravasation of medial joint fluid (*arrow*) into the reconstructed ligament (*arrowheads*).

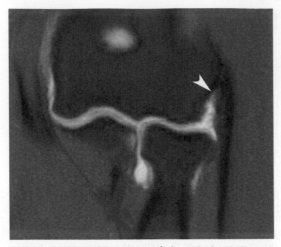

Fig. 15. High-grade tearing of the RCL in a 17-year-old boy after elbow dislocation 1 year prior. Coronal MR arthrogram shows high-grade tearing of the deep fibers of the proximal RCL (*arrowhead*), with intact overlying common extensor tendon origin. Patient also had healed coronoid process fracture (not shown).

Olecranon Stress Fracture

Osseous stress reaction, contusion, and fracture also may be detected on the fluid-sensitive sequences of elbow MR arthrography. Olecranon stress fractures in throwing athletes are caused by shear forces in the posterior compartment and chronic impingement.[1] Repetitive valgus elbow stress and rapid elbow extension during the late stages of throwing may result in olecranon

microtrauma. These repetitive excessive forces may lead to olecranon stress fracture, with propagation from a structural weak point in the trochlear groove.[35] MR imaging is reserved for cases in which radiographs are inconclusive: injected contrast may extend into portions of incomplete fractures (**Fig. 16**) and associated bone marrow edema will be evident on fluid-sensitive sequences. Initial treatment of olecranon stress fractures is conservative and consists of rest and splinting. Screw fixation may be preferable so as to achieve early union in elite athletes and hasten return to play.[36,37]

Osteochondral Injuries and Osteochondritis Dissecans

Instability of the elbow predisposes to osteochondral and articular cartilage injury; these lesions are optimally evaluated with MR arthrography, as this carries greater sensitivity than routine MR imaging or CT arthrography.[5] Arthrographic evaluation of osteochondral injury is crucial for determining the stability of these lesions, which will determine if surgical intervention is required. Along the same disease spectrum, the presence of intra-articular bodies can be much better demonstrated with MR arthrography than with conventional imaging, as the insinuation of contrast between the fragment and adjacent bone greatly improves contrast resolution.

Osteochondritis dissecans (OCD) of the elbow is a specific manifestation of osteochondral injury seen classically in adolescent or young adult athletes, especially baseball pitchers. The characteristic distribution involves the radiocapitellar joint

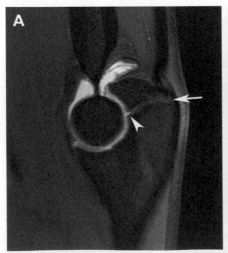
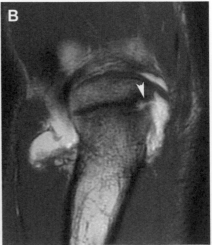

Fig. 16. Olecranon apophyseal stress fracture in a 17-year-old baseball player who also sustained partial-thickness tear of the UCL. (*A*, *B*) Sagittal T1-weighted fat-suppressed (*A*) and coronal T1-weighted (*B*) images show medial-sided stress fracture through the olecranon physis (*arrow*), with contrast extending into the medial and deep portions (*arrowheads*) of the physis.

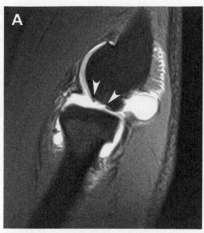
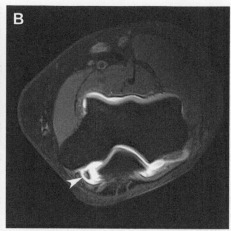

Fig. 17. OCD of the elbow. (*A*) Sagittal MR arthrographic images in a 14-year-old female athlete show a focal osteochondral defect along the articular surface of the capitellum (*white arrowheads*). (*B*) The presence of an intra-articular body (*white arrowhead*) in the olecranon recess on axial image demonstrates the end result of osteochondral instability with fragmentation.

most frequently due to repetitive valgus impaction injury of the radial head and developing ossification center of the capitellum during the late-cocking phase of pitching.[38] The pathogenesis of OCD is believed to be secondary to compromised vascular supply to the capitellum, resulting in osteochondral fragmentation and eventually, instability.[26,38] Arthrography plays a key role in determining the treatment pathway for these patients. Osteochondral injuries are visualized as irregularities along the articular surface, which fill in with intra-articular contrast.[5,38] Osteochondral instability is demonstrated by the insinuation of contrast between the fragment and underlying bone; these patients invariably require surgical repair with either pinning or excision of the osteochondral fragment. Intra-articular bodies may be present in advanced cases, and their detection is greatly improved with MR arthrography over conventional MR imaging, especially when the bodies are incompletely ossified (**Fig. 17**).[5,28,39]

SUMMARY

In conclusion, MR arthrography of the wrist and elbow is useful for detecting a variety of intra-articular pathologies, and has proven to be more sensitive and specific than conventional MR imaging. MR dictations should address whether intrinsic ligament tears of the wrist are partial-thickness or full-thickness, and involve the dorsal, membranous, and/or volar components of the ligaments. With regard to the elbow soft tissue pathology, partial-thickness tears of the anterior band of the UCL in overhead-throwing athletes are well evaluated with MR arthrography. The "T

sign" should be sought by the radiologist in cases of partial tearing at the attachment of ligament onto the sublime tubercle. Repetitive valgus elbow stress and rapid elbow extension during the late stages of throwing may result in olecranon stress fracture, with propagation from a structural weak point in the trochlear groove. And finally, MR arthrography is helpful in staging OCD of the capitellum, caused by repetitive valgus impaction injury in adolescent or young adult baseball pitchers.

REFERENCES

1. Bancroft LW. Wrist injuries: a comparison between high- and low-impact sports. Radiol Clin North Am 2013;51(2):299–311.
2. Watanabe A, Souza F, Vezeridis PS, et al. Ulnar-sided wrist pain. II. Clinical imaging and treatment. Skeletal Radiol 2010;39(9):837–57.
3. Choudur HN, Ellins ML. Ultrasound-guided gadolinium joint injections for magnetic resonance arthrography. J Clin Ultrasound 2011;39(1):6–11.
4. Medverd JR, Pugsley JM, Harley JD, et al. Lateral approach for radiocarpal wrist arthrography. AJR Am J Roentgenol 2011;196(1):W58–60.
5. Delport AG, Zoga AC. MR and CT arthrography of the elbow. Semin Musculoskelet Radiol 2012;16(1):15–26.
6. DeFilippo M, Pogliacomi F, Bertellini A, et al. MDCT arthrography of the wrist: diagnostic accuracy and indications. Eur J Radiol 2010;74:221–5.
7. Daley EL, Bajaj S, Bisson LJ, et al. Improving injection accuracy of the elbow, knee, and shoulder: does injection site and imaging make a difference? A systematic review. Am J Sports Med 2011;39(3):656–62.

8. Saupe N, Zanetti M, Pfirrmann CW, et al. Pain and other side effects after MR arthrography: prospective evaluation in 1085 patients. Radiology 2009; 250(3):830–8.

9. Squires JH, England E, Mehta K, et al. The role of imaging in diagnosing diseases of the distal radioulnar joint, triangular fibrocartilage complex, and distal ulna. AJR Am J Roentgenol 2014;203(1): 146–53.

10. Chhabra A, Soldatos T, Thawait GK, et al. Current perspectives on the advantages of 3-T MR imaging of the wrist. Radiographics 2012;32(3):879–96.

11. Donati OF, Nordmeyer-Massner J, Nanz D, et al. Direct MR arthrography of cadaveric wrists: comparison between MR imaging at 3.0T and 7.0T and gross pathologic inspection. J Magn Reson Imaging 2011;34(6):1333–40.

12. Scheck RK, Kubitzek C, Hierner R, et al. The scapholunate interosseous ligament in MR arthrography of the wrist: correlation with non-enhanced MRI and wrist arthroscopy. Skeletal Radiol 1997; 26:263–71.

13. Ringler MD. MRI of wrist ligaments. J Hand Surg Am 2013;38(10):2034–46.

14. Cerny M, Marlois R, Theumann N, et al. 3-T direct MR arthrography of the wrist: value of finger trap distraction to assess intrinsic ligament and triangular fibrocartilage complex tears. Eur J Radiol 2013; 82(10):e582–9.

15. Kirchgesner T, Pesquer L, Larbi A, et al. Axial traction in magnetic resonance arthrography of the wrist: How to do? Diagn Interv Imaging 2014 [pii:S2211-5684(14) 00194–6]. [Epub ahead of print].

16. Garcia-Elias M, Geissler WB. Carpal instability. In: Green DP, Hotchkiss RN, Pederson WC, et al, editors. Green's operative hand surgery. Philadelphia: Elsevier Churchill Livingstone; 2005. p. 535–604.

17. Cerezal L, de Dios Berná-Mestre J, Canga A, et al. MR and CT arthrography of the wrist. Semin Musculoskelet Radiol 2012;16(1):27–41.

18. Lee RK, Ng AW, Tong CS, et al. Intrinsic ligament and triangular fibrocartilage complex tears of the wrist: comparison of MDCT arthrography, conventional 3-T MRI, and MR arthrography. Skeletal Radiol 2013;42(9):1277–85.

19. Lee YH, Choi YR, Kim S, et al. Intrinsic ligament and triangular fibrocartilage complex (TFCC) tears of the wrist: comparison of isovolumetric 3D-THRIVE sequence MR arthrography and conventional MR image at 3 T. Magn Reson Imaging 2013;31(2): 221–6.

20. Moser T, Khoury V, Harris PG, et al. MDCT arthrography or MR arthrography for imaging the wrist joint? Semin Musculoskelet Radiol 2009;13(1):39–54.

21. Porteous R, Harish S, Parasu N. Imaging of ulnar-sided wrist pain. Can Assoc Radiol J 2012;63(1): 18–29.

22. Mak WH, Szabo RM, Myo GK. Assessment of volar radiocarpal ligaments: MR arthrographic and arthroscopic correlation. AJR Am J Roentgenol 2012; 198(2):423–7.

23. Taljanovic MS, Malan JJ, Sheppard JE. Normal anatomy of the extrinsic capsular wrist ligaments by 3-T MRI and high-resolution ultrasonography. Semin Musculoskelet Radiol 2012;16(2):104–14.

24. Muminagic S, Kapidzic T. Wrist instability after injury. Mater Sociomed 2012;24(2):121–4.

25. Magee T. Comparison of 3-T MRI and arthroscopy of intrinsic wrist ligament and TFCC tears. AJR Am J Roentgenol 2009;192(1):80–5.

26. Dewan AK, Chhabra AB, Khanna AJ, et al. MRI of the elbow: techniques and spectrum of disease: AAOS exhibit selection. J Bone Joint Surg Am 2013;95(14):e99, 1–13.

27. Lohman M, Borrero C, Casagranda B, et al. The posterior transtriceps approach for elbow arthrography: a forgotten technique? Skeletal Radiol 2009;38(5): 513–6.

28. Lomasney LM, Choi H, Jayanthi N. Magnetic resonance arthrography of the upper extremity. Radiol Clin North Am 2013;51(2):227–37.

29. Schaeffeler C, Waldt S, Woertler K. Traumatic instability of the elbow - anatomy, pathomechanisms and presentation on imaging. Eur Radiol 2013;23(9): 2582–93.

30. Sanal HT, Chen L, Haghighi P, et al. Annular ligament of the elbow: MR arthrography appearance with anatomic and histologic correlation. AJR Am J Roentgenol 2009;193(2):W122–6.

31. Anderson MW, Alford BA. Overhead throwing injuries of the shoulder and elbow. Radiol Clin North Am 2010;48(6):1137–54.

32. Schwartz ML, Al-Zahrani S, Morwessel RM, et al. Ulnar collateral ligament injury in the throwing athlete: Evaluation with saline-enhanced MR arthrography. Radiology 1995;197:297–9.

33. Wear SA, Thornton DD, Schwartz ML, et al. MRI of the reconstructed ulnar collateral ligament. AJR Am J Roentgenol 2011;197(5):1198–204.

34. Jacobson JA, Chiavaras MM, Lawton JM, et al. Radial collateral ligament of the elbow: sonographic characterization with cadaveric dissection correlation and magnetic resonance arthrography. J Ultrasound Med 2014;33(6):1041–8.

35. Blake JJ, Block JJ, Hannah GA, et al. Unusual stress fracture in an adolescent baseball pitcher affecting the trochlear groove of the olecranon. Pediatr Radiol 2008;38:788–90.

36. Sheehan SE, Dyer GS, Sodisckson AD, et al. Traumatic elbow injuries: what the orthopedic surgeon wants to know. RadioGraphics 2013;33:869–88.

37. Rauck RC, Lamont LE, Doyle SM. Pediatric upper extremity stress injuries. Curr Opin Pediatr 2013; 25(1):40–5.

38. Ruchelsman DE, Hall MP, Youm T. Osteochondritis dissecans of the capitellum: current concepts. J Am Acad Orthop Surg 2010;18(9): 557–67.

39. Theodoropoulos JS, Dwyer T, Wolin PM. Correlation of preoperative MRI and MRA with arthroscopically proven articular cartilage lesions of the elbow. Clin J Sport Med 2012;22(5):403–7.

MR Imaging of Soft-Tissue Tumors of the Upper Extremity

Shuji Nagata, MD, PhD[a],*, Hiroshi Nishimura, MD, PhD[b], Toshi Abe, MD, PhD[a]

KEYWORDS

- Upper extremity • Soft-tissue tumor • Benign • Malignancy • MR imaging

KEY POINTS

- Magnetic resonance (MR) imaging can definitively diagnose lipomas, neural fibrolipomas, palmar fibromatosis, benign peripheral nerve sheath tumors, and glomus tumors.
- In most benign soft-tissue tumors of the upper extremity, characteristic MR imaging features combined with clinical history and epidemiologic knowledge can predict specific diagnoses.
- Epithelloid sarcomas are rare malignant soft-tissue tumors that usually occur in the hand or forearm with lymphadenopathy.

INTRODUCTION

The most frequently encountered tumors of the upper extremity often appear elsewhere in the body. There are some lesions, however, that appear primarily in the upper extremity.

MR imaging has become the technique of choice for detecting and characterizing soft-tissue masses. Its improved soft-tissue contrast has provided significant advantages for assessing lesion conspicuity as well as characterizing the lesions and local staging. Tumors involving the upper extremity are often benign, and MR imaging can be fairly specific in diagnoses. This report provides an MR imaging review and pictorial for common soft-tissue tumors of the upper extremity.

IMAGING PROTOCOL

Evaluation of the upper extremity with MR imaging begins with proper patient positioning to maximize comfort and thereby minimize motion. The patient's arms should be placed at the isocenter of the magnet to avoid degrading signal to noise

and field homogeneity, which affects image quality. It may be useful to place a marker over the area of clinical concern, particularly with subcutaneous lipomas or small soft-tissue tumors. All efforts should be made to maximize signal to noise ratios, regardless of system design.

The field of view should be tailored to the size of both the patient and the suspected mass. Lesion size also dictates whether use of a local surface or cylindrical coil is appropriate, particularly for small lesions. Proper coil use makes it possible to image small or superficially located soft-tissue masses. Slice thickness can also vary based on the lesion.

Lesions should be imaged in at least 2 orthogonal planes, using conventional T1-weighted (T1W) and T2-weighted (T2W) spin-echo MR imaging in at least 1 plane. Because radiologists are most familiar with conventional axial anatomy, axial T1W and T2W imaging should be obtained in almost all cases. The choice of additional imaging planes vary based on the involved body part, lesion location, and relationship of the lesion to crucial structures.

The authors have nothing to disclose.
[a] Department of Radiology, Kurume University School of Medicine, 67 Asahi-machi, Kurume, Fukuoka 830-0011, Japan; [b] Department of Radiology, Saiseikai Futsukaichi Hospital, 3-13-1 Yu-machi, Chikushino, Fukuoka 818-0058, Japan
* Corresponding author.
E-mail address: sn4735@med.kurume-u.ac.jp

Magn Reson Imaging Clin N Am 23 (2015) 457–468
http://dx.doi.org/10.1016/j.mric.2015.04.002
1064-9689/15/$ – see front matter © 2015 Elsevier Inc. All rights reserved.

Fat-suppressed T2W imaging increases lesion to background signal intensity differences. It is also useful for decreasing or eliminating the MR signal from fat, allowing increased conspicuity of lesions containing paramagnetic substances, such as methemoglobin, on T1W images, and identifying contrast enhancement. Gradient-echo imaging may be a useful supplement in demonstrating hemosiderin because of its greater magnetic susceptibility. Intravenous contrast is often not required. However, it is helpful to differentiate cysts from solid masses and soft-tissue sarcomas from peripheral nonneoplastic areas of edema. Diffusion-weighted images (DWIs) provide molecular information regarding fluid motion in tissues. Apparent diffusion coefficient values calculated quantitatively from DWIs have been explored to improve lesion characterization and evaluate response to therapy. They can be performed quickly, do not require administration of exogenous contrast medium, and do not involve a significant increase in examination time.

BENIGN SOFT-TISSUE TUMORS
Lipoma

Lipomas are the most common soft-tissue neoplasm and represent about 50% of all soft-tissue tumors.[1] They can occur superficially or deeply in subcutaneous fat, muscles, synovium, or parosteal areas. Although intramuscular lipomas arise within muscle, they may involve both muscular and intermuscular tissue rather than the intermuscular region only. Intramuscular lipomas occur in patients of all ages, with most presenting between 30 and 60 years of age.[2] There is a slight male predominance. Lesions commonly affect large muscles of the lower extremity (45%), trunk (17%), shoulder (12%), and upper extremity (10%).[3]

Depending on the size and location of the intramuscular lipoma, radiography may reveal an intramuscular mass of fat density. Murphey and colleagues[3] reported that radiologic evaluation is diagnostic in up to 71% of cases. The lesion may be identified on MR images as a predominantly fatty mass with signal intensity equal to that of subcutaneous fat (**Fig. 1**). Although the mass is usually well defined and sharply circumscribed, it may have irregular margins that interdigitate with adjacent skeletal muscle. Such lesions are referred to as infiltrating lipomas.

Neural Fibrolipoma

Neural fibrolipomas are also known as fibrolipomatous hamartomas of the nerve, perineural lipomas, fatty infiltration of the nerve, and intraneural lipomas. Patients with neural fibromas typically present during early adulthood with a soft, slowly enlarging mass in the volar aspect of the hand, wrist, or forearm.[4] Approximately 80% of upper extremity lesions originate in the median nerve.[5] The lower extremity is involved less frequently. The lesion is typically present at birth or presents within the first 2 years of life.[5] Neural fibrolipomas associated with macrodactyly are known as macrodystrophia lipomatosa (**Fig. 2**).

The affected nerve is diffusely enlarged, with the epineurium and perineurium infiltrated by fibroadipose tissue that surrounds and separates normal-appearing fascicles.[6] The MR appearance of neural fibrolipomas is pathognomonic. Low signal intensity nerve bundles surrounded by increased signal intensity related to fat appear

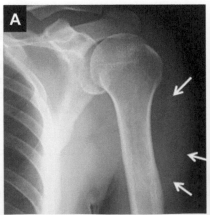
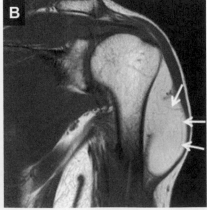

Fig. 1. Intramuscular lipoma of the left upper arm in a 56-year-old man. (*A*) Radiograph shows a radiolucent soft-tissue mass (*arrows*). (*B*) Coronal T1W image reveals the mass, with isointensity relative to subcutaneous fat within the deltoid muscle and containing thin delicate septa (*arrows*).

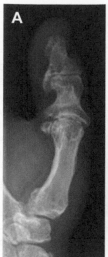
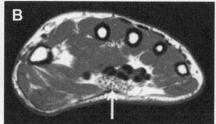
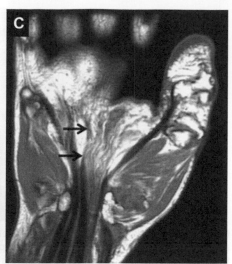

Fig. 2. Macrodystrophia lipomatosa in a 27-year-old woman. (*A*) Radiograph shows regional osseous gigantism in the first digit. (*B*) Low-signal-intensity nerve bundles surrounded by increased signal intensity related to fat appear cablelike on axial T1W image (*arrow*). (*C*) Coronal T1W image shows spaghettilike, serpentiform median nerve fascicles surrounded by fibrofatty tissue within an expanded nerve sheath (*arrows*). Cablelike and spaghettilike appearances are characteristic of neural fibrolipomas.

cablelike on axial T1W images and spaghettilike on coronal T1W images.

Angiolipoma

Angiolipomas are typically subcutaneous nodules consisting of mature fat cells intermingled with small, thin-walled capillary-type vessels, several of which contain fibrin thrombi.[7] They most commonly affect young male patients between 10 and 30 years of age. The most frequent site of involvement is the forearm, followed by the trunk and upper arm. Multiple lesions are seen in approximately 70% of cases.[3]

Areas of low signal intensity on T1W images and high signal intensity on T2W images represent vascular components enhanced with intravenous contrast material.[3] MR imaging helps discriminate between lipomas and angiolipomas that show intense enhancement on contrast-enhanced T1W images (**Fig. 3**).[8]

Nodular Fasciitis

Nodular fasciitis is a benign proliferative lesion of fibroblasts that most commonly develops at the superficial fascia in subcutaneous tissue. It is also frequently seen in intramuscular or intermuscular regions (**Fig. 4**). Lesions tend to occur between 20 and 40 years of age, growing rather rapidly with slight tenderness. They appear most often in the forearm, followed by the thigh and upper arm.

Nodular fasciitis appears round or oval and is usually well circumscribed. The lesion may be

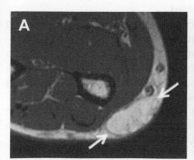
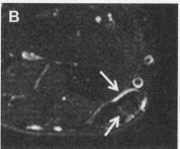
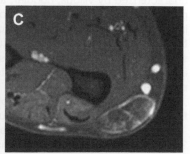

Fig. 3. Angiolipoma of the left subcutaneous forearm in a 65-year-old man. (*A*) Axial T1W image shows an encapsulated mass that is largely isointense relative to subcutaneous fat (*arrows*). The capsule and septa (*arrows*) show high signal intensity (*B*) on STIR image, which are also enhanced as a blush of small vessels (*C*) on contrast-enhanced fat-suppressed T1W image.

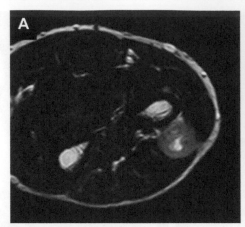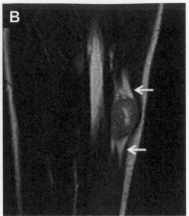

Fig. 4. Intermuscular nodular fasciitis of the left forearm in a 31-year-old man. (*A*) Axial and (*B*) sagittal T2W images show a central hyperintense mass with peripheral intermediate signal intensity representing the inverted target sign. Sagittal T2W image demonstrates a reticulated perilesional edema (*arrows*).

categorized as myxoid, cellular, or fibrous, according to predominant histologic features.[9] This histologic diversity accounts for the variable MR images of the lesions. The signal of cellular lesions appears nearly isointense to skeletal muscle on T1W images and hyperintense to that of adipose tissue on T2W images. Highly fibrous lesions have a hypointense signal on all types of MR images. The inverted target sign of a central high T2 signal with corresponding secondary to internal cystic change or necrosis is often seen.[10] Contrast enhancement is typically diffuse but may be peripheral in lesions with a greater extracellular myxoid matrix and central fluid-filled spaces.[11] An important diagnostic feature on MR imaging is linear extension of the lesion along the fascia (fascial tail appearance), which may also be enhanced with contrast.[12]

Pigmented Villonodular Synovitis

Pigmented villonodular synovitis (PVNS) represents a benign, hypertrophic synovial process characterized by villous, nodular, and villonodular proliferation and pigmentation from hemosiderin.[13] The localized extra-articular form of PVNS is frequently referred to as giant cell tumor of tendon sheath (GCTTS). Localized disease affecting an intra-articular location is referred to as the localized PVNS.

Diffuse types include conventional (or diffuse) PVNS and diffuse-type giant cell tumor (**Table 1**).

GCTTS occurs at any age with peak incidence at 20 to 40 years of age. Three-fourths of incidences occur in the digits, particularly the fingers and often on volar surfaces. There is no difference in incidence with regard to sex or ethnicity. GCTTS is generally indolent and successfully treated by

simple excision, but recurs approximately 25% of the time.[14]

MR imaging of GCTTS typically demonstrates a well-circumscribed, soft-tissue mass adjacent to the involved tendon. It shows low to intermediate signal intensity on T1W and T2W images due to hemosiderin from chronic hemorrhage, which exerts a paramagnetic effect. On gradient-echo sequences, the paramagnetic effect of hemosiderin is further exaggerated, resulting in areas of very low signal due to the blooming artifact, which is a highly suggestive feature (**Fig. 5**). The extent of enhancement of GCTTS after intravenous administration of gadolinium varies.

Fibroma of Tendon Sheath

Fibromas of the tendon sheath (FTS) is a benign fibroblastic nodular neoplasm, usually attached to a tendon sheath and also known as tenosynovial fibromas. They can occur at any age and seem to have a slight male predominance. The thumb, index, and middle fingers are most frequently involved.

On T1W images, FTSs are isointense compared with muscle, whereas signal intensity on T2W images is more variable and can range from low to high. Signal intensity on gradient-echo images is not markedly low in FST, unlike in GCTTS, because there is no hemosiderin content. Marked enhancement does not preclude a diagnosis of FTS, but lack of enhancement or mild enhancement makes FTS more likely than GCTTS (**Fig. 6**).[15]

Palmar Fibromatosis

Palmar fibromatosis is a superficial fibromatosis that represents fibroblastic and myofibroblastic

Table 1
Findings on soft-tissue tumors of the upper extremity

Diagnosis	Predilection Sites	Peak Age	Sex	Imaging Findings
Intramuscular lipoma	Extremity, trunk, shoulder	30–60 y	M > F	Interdigitate with the adjacent skeletal muscle
Neural fibrolipoma	Median nerve	10–40 y	M > F, with macrodactyly; M < F, without macrodactyly	Cablelike and spaghettilike appearance on T1WI
Angiolipoma	Forearm, trunk, upper arm	10–30 y	M > F	High signal intensity on T2WI represents vascular components enhanced on contrast-enhanced T1WI
Nodular fasciitis	Forearm, thigh, upper arm	20–40 y	M = F	Inverted target or fascial tail appearance on T2WI
GCTTS	Finger	20–40 y	M = F	Blooming artifact on gradient-echo sequences
FTS	Finger	Any age	M > F	Not markedly low signal intensity on gradient-echo sequences; lack or mild enhancement
Palmar fibromatosis	Palmar	Older than 65 y	M > F	Well-defined or ill-defined superficial mass occurring along the deep palmar aponeurosis
Neurofibroma	Skin, where the tumors are associated with small nerves	20–30 y	M = F	Target sign, centrally entering and exiting nerve signs are more common than in schwannoma
Schwannoma	Skin and subcutaneous tissue of the head, neck, and extremity	30–60 y	M = F	Peripherally entering and exiting nerve signs and cystic area are more common than in neurofibroma
Extraskeletal chondroma	Finger, hand, toe, foot	30–60 y	M > F	Mineralization characteristic of cartilaginous tumors
Glomus tumor	Finger nail bed	20–40 y	M < F	A small mass related to the nail bed with prominent and diffuse enhancement
Angioleiomyoma	Extremity	30–60 y	M < F	Either homogeneous or heterogeneous isointensity compared on T1WI and hyperintensity with few low-signal-intensity foci on T2WI, flow voids
Pilomatoricoma	Subcutaneous tissue of the head, neck, and upper extremity	<20 y	M = F	Well-circumscribed lesion with sandlike calcifications on radiography
Synovial sarcoma	Lower extremity	15–35 y	M = F	Calcification, fluid-fluid levels, triple signal intensity
Epithelioid sarcoma	Hand, forearm	10–35 y	M > F	Spread along tendon sheaths and aponeuroses

Abbreviations: FTS, fibroma of tendon sheath; T1WI, T1-weighted imaging; T2WI, T2-weighted imaging.

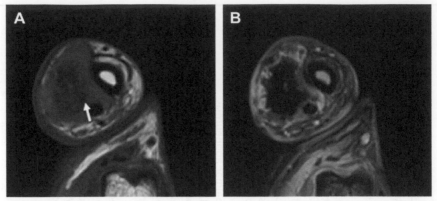

Fig. 5. Giant cell tumor of tendon sheath of the first digit in a 50-year-old woman. (*A*) Axial T1W image shows a well-circumscribed and lobulated mass abutting on the flexor tendon of the first digit (*arrow*). (*B*) Axial T2W gradient-echo image reveals accentuation (blooming) of very low signal intensity from hemosiderin deposition.

neoplasms. It most commonly occurs in patients older than 65 years, is 3 to 4 times more common in men, and is most frequent among northern Europeans.[16] Palmar fibromatosis may progress slowly to fibrous cords or bands that attach to and cause traction on the underlying flexor tendons, resulting in flexion contractures of the digits (Dupuytren contracture).

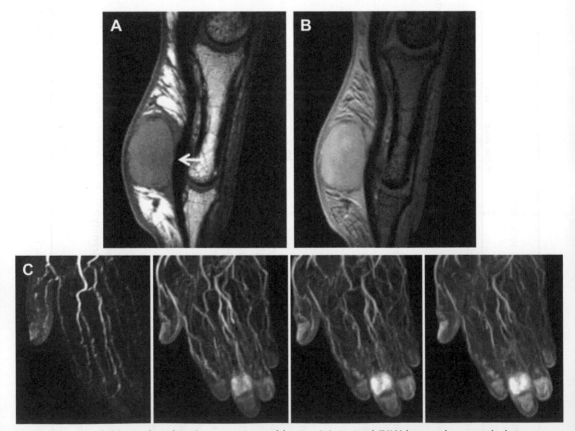

Fig. 6. Fibroma of the tendon sheath in a 56-year-old man. (*A*) Sagittal T1W image shows an isointense mass abutting on the flexor tendon of the third digit (*arrow*). (*B*) There is no blooming artifact to represent hemosiderin on sagittal T2W gradient-echo image. (*C*) Three-dimensional MR angiography demonstrates a gradual increase of enhancement. Signal intensity on the gradient-echo image and mild enhancement makes a fibroma of the tendon sheath more likely than a giant cell tumor of the tendon sheath.

The typical MR appearance of plantar fibromatosis is either a well-defined or ill-defined superficial soft-tissue mass along the palmar aponeurosis (**Fig. 7**).[17] Lesions are heterogeneous, with a signal intensity similar to that of muscle on T1W images or slightly hyperintense to muscle on T2W images. Enhancement is variable, with approximately 60% showing marked enhancement.[18]

Benign Peripheral Nerve Sheath Tumors

Benign peripheral nerve sheath tumors are divided into 2 major categories, neurofibromas and schwannomas. Pathologically, the presence of encapsulation and 2 types of Antoni areas, as well as uniformly intense immunostaining for S-100 protein, distinguish a schwannoma from a neurofibroma.

Neurofibromas most frequently affect patients between 20 and 30 years of age and represent slightly greater than 5% of benign soft-tissue neoplasms.[19] Most lesions are solitary, but up to 10% are associated with neurofibromatosis type 1. Neurofibromas are intimately associated with the parent nerve, growing in a longitudinal fusiform manner.

Schwannomas are well-encapsulated tumors that arise from Schwann cells of the nerve sheath and are also known as neurilemmomas and neurinomas. They are composed of a highly ordered cellular component (Antoni A area) and a loose myxoid component (Antoni B area). Greater than 90% of the lesions are solitary and sporadic, affect all ages, and have a peak incidence between 30 and 60 years of age. There is no known predisposition with regard to race or gender.[20] Common sites of involvement include cutaneous nerves in the head, neck, and flexor surface of the extremities.

A target sign and centrally entering and exiting nerve sign are more common in neurofibromas (58% and 42%, respectively) than in schwannomas (15% and 23%, respectively), whereas peripherally entering and exiting nerve sign and a cystic area are more common in schwannomas (77% and 64%, respectively) than in neurofibromas (58% and 38%, respectively) (**Fig. 8**).[21]

Extraskeletal Chondroma

Extraskeletal chondromas are benign cartilaginous tumors with no connection to the underlying bone and are also known as soft-tissue chondromas and chondromas of the soft part. The tumor mainly affects adults between 30 and 60 years of age and is rare in children.[22,23] Men are affected more frequently than women. Two-thirds of tumors occur on the fingers, whereas the remainder arises on the hands, followed by the toes and feet.

Mineralization of hyaline cartilage typically has a ringlike, punctate, or granular appearance characteristic of cartilaginous tumors. However, tumors sometimes present variable noncharacteristic mineralization.[24] Extraskeletal chondromas show as high signal intensity on T2W images, related to the high water content of hyaline cartilage (**Fig. 9**).

Glomus Tumor

Glomus tumors are neoplasms that develop from the neuromyoarterial glomus body. The most common location is the subungual area of digits, followed by the palm, wrist, forearm, and foot. Glomus tumors have no gender predilection, although there is a 3:1 female predominance for subungual lesions.[25] Lesions are most frequently diagnosed between 20 and 40 years of age. The classic clinical triad of pain, point tenderness,

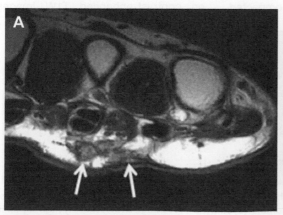
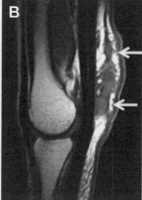

Fig. 7. Palmar fibromatosis in a 53-year-old woman with digit contractures. (*A*) Axial T2W and (*B*) sagittal T1W images show slightly hyperintense superficial bands (*arrows*) that cause flexion contractures because of their attachment to flexor tendons.

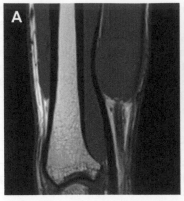
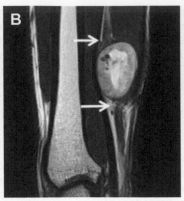
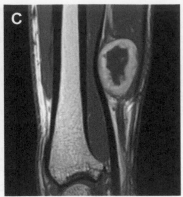

Fig. 8. Schwannoma of the median nerve in a 27-year-old man. (A) Sagittal T1W image shows that the mass is homogeneously isointense relative to muscle. (B) Sagittal T2W image shows high signal intensity with a very-high-signal-intensity central region, representing cystic change. The median nerve is eccentric in relation to the mass and shows entering and exiting nerve sign (arrows). (C) Contrast-enhanced T1W image demonstrates enhancement without a central cystic region.

and cold sensitivity is present in approximately 30% of cases.[26]

MR images show a small mass related to the nail bed, with intermediate to low signal intensity on T1W images and homogeneous high signal intensity on T2W images. A high-resolution surface coil can help detect the tumor and cortical bone erosion (Fig. 10). Enhancement is typically prominent and diffuse. Three-dimensional contrast-enhanced MR angiography is useful for precisely identifying the location and extension of tumors (see Fig. 10).

Angioleiomyoma

Angioleiomyomas, also known as a vascular leiomyomas, are common benign tumors composed of mature smooth muscle bundles surrounding vascular channels. The tumors are histopathologically subdivided into 3 types. The solid type is composed of small vessels and compacted smooth muscle, the venous type has numerous thick-walled vessels and smooth muscle bundles that are not as compact, and the cavernous type has dilated vessels and few intervening smooth muscle cells. Tumors are most frequently found in women between 30 and 60 years of age and usually occur in an extremity. Tenderness and pain, often paroxysmal and precipitated by light touch or changes in temperature, are presenting features in 50% to 70% of cases.[27,28]

The lesion signal appears with either homogeneous or heterogeneous isointensity compared with muscle on T1W images and mainly hyperintensity with few low-signal-intensity foci on T2W images. The smooth muscle cells and patent vessels are thought to correspond to hyperintense areas, whereas the low-signal-intensity foci correlate with fibrous tissue or intravascular thrombi within the mass.[29] Hyperintense signal areas on T2W images show strong enhancement on contrast-enhanced T1W images, whereas

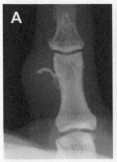
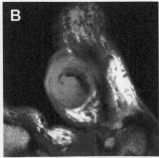
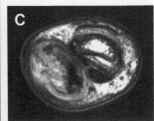

Fig. 9. Extraskeletal chondroma of the right first digit in a 64-year-old man. (A) Radiograph shows a soft-tissue mass with calcification typical of cartilage tumors. (B) Sagittal T1W image shows slightly high signal intensity relative to muscle with low signal intensity corresponding to the calcification. (C) The mass shows heterogeneously high signal intensity on axial T2W image. There is a small area of cortical attachment to the volar aspect of the phalanx without corticomedullary continuity.

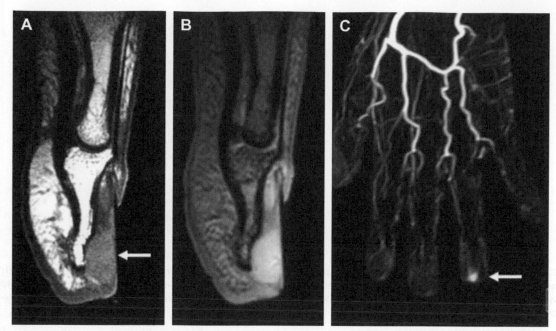

Fig. 10. Glomus tumor in a 50-year-old woman with left fourth digit pain. (*A*) Sagittal T1W image shows a slightly hyperintense tumor on the nail bed, with bone erosion (*arrow*). (*B*) The tumor shows homogeneously high signal intensity on sagittal T2W image. (*C*) Arterial phase of 3-dimensional MR angiography demonstrates avid contrast enhancement (*arrow*).

low-signal-intensity foci on T2W images enhance less.[30] Flow voids are frequently evident within the tumor (**Fig. 11**).

Pilomatricoma

Pilomatricomas are rare, benign dermal or subcutaneous tumors originating in the hair matrix and are also known as calcifying epitheliomas and pilomatrixomas. They are usually confined to subcutaneous tissue and located in the head, neck, and upper extremity. Intracellular and stromal calcification is reported in about 70% of cases, and tumors with large areas or nests of shadow cells proportionally have increased calcium deposition.[31] Most tumors arise in people younger than 20 years, although a second peak of occurrence is seen in older patients.[32] They are usually painless, slow-growing, hard masses.

Radiologic findings for a pilomatricoma typically demonstrate a well-circumscribed lesion with sand-like calcifications on plain radiography and computerized tomography. It shows inhomogeneous low signal intensity on T2W images (**Fig. 12**). Peripheral enhancement of connective tissue and/or patchy or reticular central enhancement of intercellular stroma on contrast-enhanced T1W images are characteristic.[33,34]

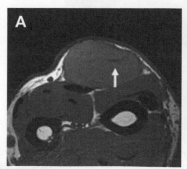
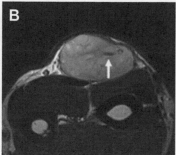
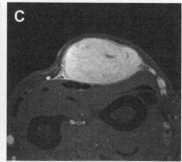

Fig. 11. Angioleiomyoma of the right forearm in a 26-year-old man. The tumor in subcutaneous fat shows isointensity relative to muscle (*A*) on T1W image and high signal intensity (*B*) on T2W image. A flow void is seen within the mass on both images (*arrow*). (*C*) Contrast-enhanced fat-suppressed T1W image demonstrates avid enhancement.

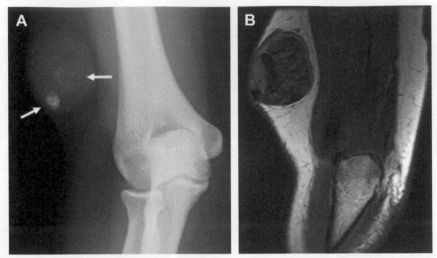

Fig. 12. Pilomatricoma of the right upper arm in a 43-year-old man. (*A*) Radiograph shows a soft-tissue mass with amorphous calcifications (*arrows*). (*B*) Sagittal T2W image demonstrates a well-defined mass located entirely within a subcutaneous fat layer and widely abutting on the skin. The mass shows heterogeneously multiple hypointense areas corresponding to calcifications.

MALIGNANT SOFT-TISSUE TUMORS
Synovial Sarcoma

Synovial sarcomas account for approximately 10% of all soft-tissue sarcomas. Although the tumor resembles synovium under light microscopy, its origin is likely from undifferentiated mesenchymal tissue. These tumors typically occur in adults between 15 and 35 years of age in the soft tissues of the extremities, particularly around large

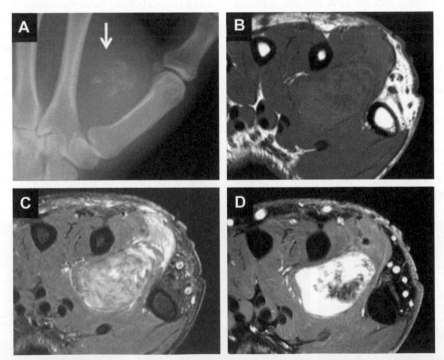

Fig. 13. Synovial sarcoma of the left hand in a 16-year-old boy. (*A*) Radiograph shows a soft-tissue mass containing calcifications (*arrow*) between the first and second metacarpals. The mass continues to abut the base of the second metacarpal along the volar aspect without definite evidence for underlying cortical involvement on (*B*) axial T1W and (*C*) fat-suppressed T2W images. Areas of decreased signal centrally within the mass on both images are compatible with calcifications seen on radiographs. (*D*) The contrast-enhanced fat-suppressed T1W image shows avid enhancement without calcifications.

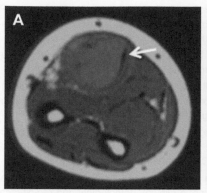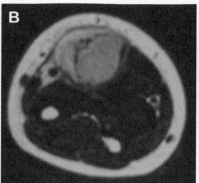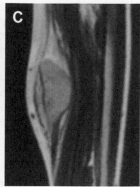

Fig. 14. Epithelioid sarcoma of the left forearm in an 8-year-old girl. (*A*) Axial T1W image shows a slightly hyperintense mass superficial to the flexor carpi radialis muscle. The tendon of the flexor digitorum superficialis (*arrow*) is involved with the mass. (*B*) Axial and (*C*) sagittal T2W images show high signal intensity.

joints, with two-thirds arising in the lower extremity.[35] The tumors occur in the upper extremity in roughly 13% of cases.

Radiographs demonstrate calcification in 20% to 30% of synovial sarcomas (**Fig. 13**A).[36] The tumor typically appears as a multilobulated soft tissue mass with similar intensity to or slightly higher intensity than that of muscle on T1W images and prominently heterogeneous high intensity on T2W images (**Fig. 13**B, C). Fluid-fluid levels due to intratumoral hemorrhage are present in almost one-fifth of cases. Mixed areas of hyperintensity, isointensity, and hypointensity relative to fat, referred to as triple signal intensity, are seen on T2W images for 35% of cases.[35] Contrast-enhanced T1W images typically demonstrate prominent and heterogeneous enhancement (**Fig. 13**D). Synovial sarcomas with a diameter less than 5 cm may have a more benign appearance, with well-circumscribed margins and homogeneous high signal intensity on T2W images.[37]

Epithelioid Sarcoma

Epithelioid sarcomas usually occur in the distal parts of extremities, particularly the hands and forearm, and have a propensity to spread along tendon sheaths and aponeuroses. Patients may also demonstrate palpable lymphadenopathy in the affected extremity. The mass is most prevalent in adolescents and young adults 10 to 35 years of age. Male patients outnumber female patients by about 2 to 1.

Calcification occurs in approximately 20% of cases.[38] The signal of the lesion on T1W images is usually isointense to that of muscle, with areas of high signal intensity caused by hemorrhage. On T2W images, signal intensity varies greatly from homogenous isointensity to heterogeneous hyperintensity, depending on hemorrhagic necrosis,

calcification, mucin, and fibrosis.[39] Peritumoral edemalike signal areas are commonly seen (**Fig. 14**).

SUMMARY

Various soft-tissue tumors arise from the upper extremity. Some have characteristic imaging features detected by radiography and MR imaging. This information, with clinical history and epidemiologic knowledge, can be used to reliably predict a specific diagnosis.

REFERENCES

1. Myhre-Jensen O. A consecutive 7-year series of 1331 benign soft tissue tumors. Clinicopathologic data. Comparison with sarcomas. Acta Orthop Scand 1981;52:287–93.
2. Weiss SW, Goldblum JR, Enzinger FM. Enzinger and Weiss's soft tissue tumors. 4th edition. St Louis (MO): Mosby; 2001.
3. Murphey MD, Carroll JF, Flemming DJ, et al. From the archives of the AFIP: benign musculoskeletal lipomatous lesions. Radiographics 2004;24:1433–66.
4. Silverman TA, Enzinger FM. Fibrolipomatous hamartoma of nerve. A clinicopathologic analysis of 26 cases. Am J Surg Pathol 1985;9:7–14.
5. Amadio PC, Reiman HM, Dobyns JH. Lipofibromatous hamartoma of nerve. J Hand Surg Am 1988; 13:67–75.
6. Shankman S, Kolla S, Beltran J. MR imaging of tumors and tumor-like lesions of the upper extremity. Magn Reson Imaging Clin N Am 2004;12:349–59.
7. Sciot R, Mandahl N. Adipocytic tumours. In: Fletcher CD, Bridge JA, Hogendoorn PC, et al, editors. WHO classification of tumours of soft tissue and bone. Lyon (France): IARC; 2013. p. 19–43.
8. Jourjon R, Dohan A, Brouland JP, et al. Angiolipoma of the labia majora: MR imaging findings with histopathological correlation. Clin Imaging 2013;37:965–8.

9. Wang XL, De Schepper AM, Vanhoenacker F, et al. Nodular fasciitis: correlation of MRI findings and histopathology. Skeletal Radiol 2002;31:155–61.

10. Coyle J, White LM, Dickson B, et al. MRI characteristic of nodular fasciitis of the musculoskeletal system. Skeletal Radiol 2013;42:975–82.

11. Dinauer PA, Brixey CJ, Moncur JT, et al. Pathologic and MR imaging features of benign fibrous soft-tissue tumors in adults. Radiographics 2007; 27:173–87.

12. Beaman FD, Kransdorf MJ, Andrews TR, et al. Superficial soft-tissue masses: analysis, diagnosis, and differential considerations. Radiographics 2007;27:509–23.

13. Reilly KE, Stern PJ, Dale JA. Recurrent giant cell tumors of the tendon sheath. J Hand Surg Am 1999; 24:1298–302.

14. Murphey MD, Rhee JH, Lewis RB, et al. Pigmented villonodular synovitis: radiologic-pathologic correlation. Radiographics 2008;28(5):1493–518.

15. De Maeseneer M, Van Isacker T, Lenchik L, et al. Fibroma of the tendon sheath of the long head of the biceps tendon. Skeletal Radiol 2014;43:399–402.

16. Bayat A, McGrouther DA. Management of Dupuytren's disease - clear advice for an elusive condition. Ann R Coll Surg Engl 2006;88:3–8.

17. Murphey MD, Ruble CM, Tyszko SM, et al. From the archives of the AFIP: musculoskeletal fibromatoses: radiologic-pathologic correlation. Radiographics 2009;29:2143–73.

18. Morrison WB, Schweitzer ME, Wapner KL, et al. Plantar fibromatosis: a benign aggressive neoplasm with a characteristic appearance on MR images. Radiology 1994;193(3):841–5.

19. Murphey MD, Smith WS, Smith SE, et al. From the archives of the AFIP. Imaging of musculoskeletal neurogenic tumors: radiologic-pathologic correlation. Radiographics 1999;19:1253–80.

20. Antonescu CR, Perry A, Woodruff JM. Schwannoma (including variants). In: Fletcher CD, Bridge JA, Hogendoorn PC, et al, editors. WHO classification of tumours of soft tissue and bone. Lyon (France): IARC; 2013. p. 170–2.

21. Jee WH, Oh SN, McCauley T, et al. Extraaxial neurofibromas versus neurilemmomas: discrimination with MRI. AJR Am J Roentgenol 2004;183:629–33.

22. Chung EB, Enzinger FM. Chondroma of soft parts. Cancer 1978;41:1414–24.

23. Smida M, Abdenaji W, Douira-Khomsi W, et al. Childhood soft tissue chondroma. Two cases report. Tunis Med 2011;89(4):379–82.

24. Le Corroller T, Bouvier-Labin C, Champsaur P. Diffuse mineralization of forearm extraskeletal chondroma. Joint Bone Spine 2008;75:479–81.

25. Shugart RR, Soule EH, Johnson EW Jr. Glomus tumor. Surg Gynecol Obstet 1963;117:334–40.

26. Drapé JL, Idy-Peretti I, Goettmann S, et al. Subungual glomus tumors: evaluation with MR imaging. Radiology 1995;195(2):507–15.

27. Hachisuga T, Hashimoto H, Enjoji M. Angioleiomyoma. A clinicopathologic reappraisal of 562 cases. Cancer 1984;54:126–30.

28. Ramesh P, Annapureddy SR, Khan F, et al. Angioleiomyoma: a clinical, pathological and radiological review. Int J Clin Pract 2004;58:587–91.

29. Gupte C, Butt SH, Tirabosco R, et al. Angioleiomyoma: magnetic resonance imaging features in ten cases. Skeletal Radiol 2008;37(11):1003–9.

30. Yoo HJ, Choi JA, Chung JH, et al. Angioleiomyoma in soft tissue of extremities: MRI findings. AJR Am J Roentgenol 2009;192:W291–4.

31. Rotenberg M, Laccourreye O, Cauchois R, et al. Head and neck pilomatrixoma. Am J Otolaryngol 1996;17:133–5.

32. Kaddu S, Soyer HP, Cerroni L, et al. Clinical and histopathologic spectrum of pilomatricomas in adults. Int J Dermatol 1994;33:705–8.

33. Masih S, Sorenson SM, Gentili A, et al. Atypical adult non-calcified pilomatricoma. Skeletal Radiol 2000; 29:54–6.

34. Lim HW, Im SA, Lim GY, et al. Pilomatricomas in children: imaging characteristics with pathologic correlation. Pediatr Radiol 2007;37:549–55.

35. Kransdorf MJ. Malignant soft-tissue tumors in a large referral population: distribution of diagnoses by age, sex, and location. AJR Am J Roentgenol 1995;164:129–34.

36. McCarville MB, Spunt SL, Skapek SX, et al. Synovial sarcoma in pediatric patients. AJR Am J Roentgenol 2002;179:797–801.

37. Blacksin MF, Siegel JR, Benevenia J, et al. Synovial sarcoma: frequency of nonaggressive MR characteristics. J Comput Assist Tomogr 1997;21: 785–9.

38. Morel M, Taïeb S, Penel N, et al. Imaging of the most frequent superficial soft-tissue sarcomas. Skeletal Radiol 2011;40(3):271–84.

39. Hanna SL, Kaste S, Jenkins JJ, et al. Epithelioid sarcoma: clinical, MR imaging and pathologic findings. Skeletal Radiol 2002;31(7):400–12.

MR Imaging of the Nerves of the Upper Extremity
Elbow to Wrist

Benjamin Matthew Howe, MD[a],*, Robert J. Spinner, MD[b],
Joel P. Felmlee, PhD[a], Matthew A. Frick, MD[a]

KEYWORDS

• Nerve • Entrapment • MR imaging • Neuropathy • Elbow • Wrist

KEY POINTS

• A solid knowledge of nerve anatomy coupled with high-quality, standard MR sequences is a strong tool in the evaluation of patients with upper extremity neuropathies.
• Patterns of MR muscle denervation help confirm and localize nerve pathology.
• MR imaging can often confirm clinically suspected entrapment sites while excluding extrinsic masses, ganglion cysts, and variant anatomy for preoperative planning.

INTRODUCTION

The peripheral nervous system is susceptible to a diverse array of pathologic insults, which may be broadly categorized into 2 categories: those entities intrinsic to the nerves themselves, either primarily arising within the nerve(s) or direct involvement of the nerve(s) secondary to a systemic process, and processes external to the nerve(s) proper but affecting them extrinsically via mass effect, such as entrapment neuropathies. Tumors (primary and metastatic), tumorlike conditions, and inflammatory conditions may also affect peripheral nerves. Lacking the osseous protection of the spine and cranium, the peripheral nervous system is also susceptible to traumatic injury.

In the past, clinicians depended largely on combined findings from a patient's history, physical examination, and electrophysiologic testing to localize and characterize suspected peripheral neuropathies. Today's clinicians are aided greatly by the tremendous advances in cross-sectional imaging that have occurred during the past several decades. Although remarkable contributions in ultrasound technology and improved user performance contribute greatly to the current evaluation and management of peripheral neuropathies, this review focuses primarily on the use of MR imaging in the diagnosis and management of peripheral nerve disorders of the upper extremity.

The soft tissue contrast inherent to high-quality MR imaging allows for outstanding visualization of the peripheral nervous system and surrounding structures. MR imaging examinations of the peripheral nervous system should ideally be performed on a 3T magnet paired with a surface coil, which allows for imaging of the entire suspected area of abnormality. For those examinations requiring imaging of structures away from the isocenter of the magnet, use of a dedicated transmit/receive coil is of great benefit in an attempt to mitigate known artifacts that can occur in this setting.

Standard sequences should include transverse, typically axial, T1, and fat-suppressed T2-weighted images. Similarly weighted coronal and

---

The authors have nothing to disclose.
[a] Department of Radiology, Mayo Clinic, 200 First Street SW, Rochester, MN 55905, USA; [b] Department of Neurologic Surgery, Mayo Clinic, 200 First Street SW, Rochester, MN 55905, USA
* Corresponding author.
E-mail address: Howe.benjamin@mayo.edu

Magn Reson Imaging Clin N Am 23 (2015) 469–478
http://dx.doi.org/10.1016/j.mric.2015.04.009
1064-9689/15/$ – see front matter © 2015 Elsevier Inc. All rights reserved.

mri.theclinics.com

sagittal images obliquely oriented along the long axis of the fibers or course of the suspected involved nerve(s) are also of great benefit for both diagnosis, for example, appreciating caliber change in the setting of entrapment neuropathy, and treatment planning, for example, preoperative localization for biopsy and/or operative resection. The authors strongly advocate the use of gadolinium in all cases, without contraindications, presenting for MR evaluation of suspected peripheral neuropathy because some inflammatory disorders may only be appreciated as subtle enhancement on postgadolinium sequences.

The median, radial, and ulnar nerves are susceptible to entrapment at multiple well-established sites between the arm and the wrist. The anatomy of each nerve is reviewed individually followed by a discussion of known entrapment neuropathies affecting that nerve.

IMAGING OF ENTRAPMENT NEUROPATHIES

Entrapment neuropathies are common at the elbow and wrist. The most common entrapment in the upper extremity is the median nerve at the level of the carpal tunnel, followed by the ulnar nerve at the cubital tunnel. The purpose of MR imaging of entrapment neuropathy is to confirm the clinical suspicion and identify factors contributing to entrapment. Perpendicular (axial) and sagittal to the long axis of the nerve are the best planes for the evaluation of entrapment neuropathy. Axial images typically offer the best spatial resolution for evaluation of fascicular architecture. A high-resolution T1-weighted sequence is best for demonstrating the fine intrafascicular fat present in normal nerves. Peripheral nerves are surrounded typically by a thin rim of perineural fat that also may become effaced, scarred, or inflamed and edematous in the setting of entrapment neuropathies. The sagittal image plane parallel to the long axis of the nerve best depicts the location and severity of the entrapment. Fluid-sensitive sagittal sequences are most helpful in localizing the point of entrapment, because the nerves demonstrate enlargement and increased T2-weighted hyperintensity near the point of entrapment. The inflammatory response associated with entrapment, that is, neuritis, gradually decreases both proximal and distal to the point of entrapment. In severe nerve entrapments, the nerve demonstrates a decreased T2-weighted signal at the point of entrapment with increased T2-weighted signal proximal and distal to the point of compression, the so-called triple B sign of a bright, black, bright nerve.[1] In some instances, 3-dimensional isovolumetric sequences may be

helpful in obtaining true sagittal and axial planes to the nerves.

Anatomic variations are well-recognized as additional or potential factors predisposing nerve entrapment. These anatomic considerations are discussed herein as they pertain to the common entrapment sites.

IMAGING OF TUMORS AND INFLAMMATORY NEUROPATHIES

Soft tissue tumors and ganglion cysts may cause neuropathy at the elbow or wrist. Tumors and tumorlike conditions affecting peripheral nerves may be either extrinsic to the nerve (metastasis or sarcoma) or intrinsic to the nerve, as in the setting of benign and malignant peripheral nerve sheath tumors. Similarly, ganglion cysts may be either intraneural or extraneural and are an additional well-recognized cause of peripheral neuropathy. Intraneural ganglion cysts have been reported at both the elbow[2] and the wrist.[3,4] It is important to distinguish between intraneural and extraneural ganglion cysts and the joint connection for surgical planning purposes.

MR imaging is useful in the evaluation of poorly localizable peripheral nerve pathology, such as inflammatory conditions. In this clinical setting, electromyography is often performed before MR imaging and may aid in localization and thus narrow the anatomic region to be covered. Diffuse inflammatory processes typically have a nonspecific MR imaging appearance with T2-weighted hyperintensity and variable nerve enlargement. As noted, these authors advocate the use of gadolinium in MR evaluation of all suspected peripheral neuropathies in the absence of contraindications. Postgadolinium imaging with fat saturation is particularly useful in evaluation of inflammatory neuropathy because most inflammatory neuropathies demonstrate no or minimal, thin peripheral postgadolinium enhancement. Normal peripheral nerves demonstrate no postgadolinium enhancement owing to the inability of gadolinium to cross an intact blood–nerve barrier. Inflammation can disrupt the endothelial tight junctions at the blood–nerve barrier, resulting in abnormal nerve enhancement.[5,6]

Several tumorlike conditions of the peripheral nerves demonstrate relatively specific imaging findings. Chronic inflammatory polyneuropathies and mononeuropathies typically demonstrate marked fusiform nerve enlargement and T2 hyperintensity with no or minimal peripheral postgadolinium enhancement. Intraneural perineurioma is a benign lesion that typically presents in children and young adults. MR findings include fusiform enlargement, T2-weighted hyperintensity, and markedly diffuse postgadolinium enhancement of the nerve.[7] Lipomatosis of nerve (fibrolipomatous hamartoma) has characteristic MR features of nerve enlargement with increased intraneural fat. It is most common in the median nerve and can be diagnosed confidently on MR without the need for a biopsy.[8]

MEDIAN NERVE
Anatomy

The median nerve is formed by contributions from the lateral (C5, C6, and C7) and medial cords (C8 and T1). The median nerve forms in the axilla and runs in the medial arm, adjacent to the brachial artery. The nerve passes through the antebrachial fossa and travels deep to the proximal margin of the pronator teres in the proximal forearm. The anterior interosseous nerve (AIN) branches off the median nerve in the proximal forearm. In the forearm, the median nerve is located deep to the flexor carpi radialis and flexor digitorum superficialis muscles. The palmar cutaneous branch of the median nerve originates in the distal forearm before the median nerve entering the carpal tunnel. The palmar cutaneous branch supplies sensory innervation to the lateral palm over the thenar eminence and does not pass through the carpal tunnel. The carpal tunnel contains the median nerve and 9 flexor tendons (flexor digitorum superficialis, flexor digitorum profundus, and flexor pollicis longus). The median nerve branches distal to the carpal tunnel into the digital nerve branches and provides sensation to the palmar thumb, index, long, and radial half of the ring finger.

The median nerve does not provide motor innervation in the arm. Motor branches to the pronator teres, flexor carpi radialis, flexor digitorum superficialis, and palmaris longus are given off at the level of the elbow. The AIN branches from the median nerve in the proximal forearm and provides motor innervation to the deep muscles in the anterior compartment of the forearm: namely, the flexor pollicis longus, pronator quadratus, and radial aspect of the flexor digitorum profundus. Muscular branches from the median nerve provide motor innervation to all the remaining flexor compartment muscles with the exception of the flexor carpi ulnaris and a portion of the flexor digitorum profundus, both of which receive motor innervation from the ulnar nerve. The recurrent thenar branch of the median nerve supplies the thenar muscles of the hand, the first and second lumbricals, the opponens pollicis, the abductor pollicis brevis, and the flexor pollicis brevis (so-called LOAF muscles). The recurrent thenar branch has been referred to as the "million dollar branch" because inadvertent iatrogenic injury during carpal tunnel surgery may lead to significant morbidity and a subsequent lawsuit.

Pathology

Carpal tunnel syndrome
The median nerve at the carpal tunnel is the most common site of upper extremity nerve entrapment. Patients typically present with classic symptoms of median neuropathy of the hand and are most often diagnosed clinically and treated without the need for advanced imaging techniques. Any mass in the region can result in median nerve compression at the wrist/palm and can again be either intraneural or extraneural. Intraneural causes include peripheral nerve sheath tumors and lipomatous overgrowth/enlargement of nerve (fibrolipomatous hamartoma).[9,10] Extraneural causes include ganglion cysts, lipomas, heterotopic ossification, and vascular malformations, to name a few.[9,11–13] MR imaging may be particularly helpful in patients with symptoms suggestive of carpal tunnel syndrome when they have a mass lesion, in those patients with atypical presentations primarily, or in those who have not responded or recurred after primary carpal tunnel release (Fig. 1).

The pathophysiology of idiopathic carpal tunnel syndrome is not known entirely. Synovial

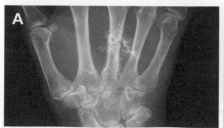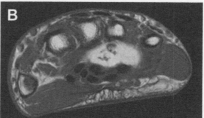

Fig. 1. Frontal radiograph of the hand in a patient with carpal tunnel syndrome demonstrates benign calcifications in the palm distal to the carpal tunnel (A). An axial T1-weighted MR imaging demonstrates an extraneural mass primarily composed of mature fat (B) with dystrophic central calcification consistent with a benign lipoma.

hypertrophy and fibrosis occurs and ultimately results in increased carpal tunnel pressure and compression of the median nerve.[14–16] The fibrosis is accompanied by vascular proliferation and hypertrophy.[16,17] When advanced, this subsynovial connective tissue fibrosis may decrease the normal gliding mechanics of the flexor tendons in the carpal tunnel that may exacerbate median nerve irritation.[18] Patients often present with classic symptoms of median neuropathy at the wrist (including paresthesias of the radial 3 $\frac{1}{2}$ digits, which are worse at night or when driving a car and improved with shaking the hand). Patients with classic symptoms are most often diagnosed on clinical grounds and treated without the need for advanced imaging techniques.

Numerous studies have evaluated the utility of MR imaging in evaluating patients with carpal tunnel syndrome. T2-weighted quantitative mapping, diffusion-weighted, and diffusion tensor sequences are advanced techniques that have been reported in the evaluation of idiopathic carpal tunnel syndrome.[19–22] MR features associated with the clinical diagnosis of carpal tunnel syndrome include thenar muscle denervation edema and/or atrophy, decreased cross-sectional diameter of the nerve in the carpal tunnel compared with diameter proximal to the tunnel, bowing of the flexor retinaculum, and hyperintensity of the nerve proximal and distal to the compression.

Anterior interosseous nerve syndrome

AIN syndrome is rare. It is not typically associated with mass effect. Although entrapment (such as by fibrous bands) has been put forth, more commonly the cause of AIN syndrome is often unknown or is of an inflammatory nature.[23] MR imaging may support the diagnosis when the characteristic pattern of muscular denervation change is present (**Fig. 2**). The AIN innervates the flexor pollicis longus, pronator quadratus, and flexor digitorum profundus of the index and middle fingers.[23,24] Isolated edema in the pronator quadratus should be interpreted with caution, because it is found commonly in asymptomatic individuals and does not necessarily indicate denervation changes.[25] In AIN syndrome the nerve typically demonstrates nonspecific T2-weighted hyperintensity.[23]

Median nerve compression in the proximal forearm

The median nerve passes between the deep and superficial heads of the pronator teres in the proximal forearm. Although rare and controversial, the median nerve may become entrapped in this region. This is known as pronator teres syndrome.[26,27] Patients present typically with aching forearm pain with tenderness to palpation or a Tinel's sign localized to the proximal margin of the pronator teres, and symptoms may increase with pronation and supination of the forearm.[26,28] An additional potential site of median nerve entrapment in the proximal forearm is at the tendinous arch between the radial and humeral heads of the flexor digitorum superficialis that is volar to the median nerve referred to as the "sublimis bridge."[28] Additional potential etiologies of compression of the median nerve in the proximal forearm include masses, accessory muscles (Gantzer's muscle, accessory head of the flexor pollicis longus), and the bicipital aponeurosis.[28–30] The ligament of Struthers and associated supracondylar process is a site of median nerve entrapment that is located above the elbow with similar clinical features as entrapment in the proximal forearm. An anatomic study by Natsis[31] found

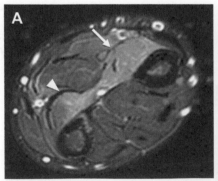 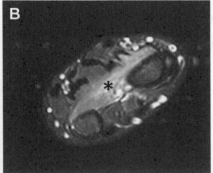

Fig. 2. Axial T2-weighted fat-saturated images of the mid (*A*) and distal forearm (*B*) in a patient with symptoms of anterior interosseous nerve syndrome. The images demonstrate the classic pattern of denervation involving the flexor digitorum profundus (*A, arrowhead*), flexor pollicis longus (*A, arrow*), and pronator quadratus (*B, asterisk*). The MR imaging did not demonstrate a mass or findings to suggest entrapment. It was felt to be inflammatory in nature. (*Courtesy of* Kimberly K. Amrami, MD, Mayo Clinic, Rochester, MN.)

that, when present, the supracondylar process located an average of 59.8 mm proximal to the medial epicondyle with 79.0 mm being the furthest location proximal to the epicondyle.

ULNAR NERVE
Anatomy

The ulnar nerve arises from the C8-T1 nerves. It descends in the posteromedial aspect of the arm. In the distal arm, it passes through the medial intramuscular septum. The nerve next passes through the cubital tunnel at the elbow. The cubital tunnel floor is osseous and formed by the posterior aspect of the medial humeral epicondyle. The roof of the tunnel is formed by a fibrous band know as Osborne's ligament. An anconeus epitrochlearis muscle reportedly is present in 11% of the population and occurs in the location of Osborne's ligament.[32,33] After the cubital tunnel, the nerve passes between the ulnar and humeral origins of the flexor carpi ulnaris. It parallels the ulnar artery in the forearm in a plane superficial to the flexor digitorum profundus and deep to the flexor digitorum superficialis and flexor carpi ulnaris. The ulnar nerve passes into Guyon's canal at the wrist. The pisiform and the hamate form the borders of the canal with the flexor retinaculum forming the floor and the volar carpal ligament forming the roof. In the distal portion of Guyon's canal, the ulnar nerve bifurcates into the deep and superficial branches.

Just distal to the elbow, the ulnar nerve provides innervation to the flexor carpi ulnaris and the flexor digitorum profundus muscle to the ring and little fingers. About 6 cm proximal to the wrist, the dorsal cutaneous nerve is given off; this provides sensation to the dorsal aspect of the hand. At the palm, the deep branch innervates the hypothenar muscles (abductor digiti minimi, flexor digiti minimi brevis, and opponens digiti minimi), the third and fourth lumbricals, and the palmar and dorsal interossei muscles. The superficial branch provides sensation to the palmar aspect of the little finger and ulnar half of the ring finger.

Pathology

Cubital tunnel syndrome
Ulnar nerve entrapment at the cubital tunnel is a common indication for upper extremity nerve imaging. MR imaging of cubital tunnel syndrome is useful for direct evaluation of the ulnar nerve for abnormality in suspected cases and in excluding variant anatomy or compressive masses or cysts. T2-weighted nerve hyperintensity and increased nerve size are found in symptomatic patients[34–37]; however, Husarik and colleagues[38] evaluated the nerves about the elbow in 60 asymptomatic patients and found that 60% had increased T2-weighted ulnar nerve signal in the cubital tunnel. MR imaging is useful in determining additional factors that may be contributing to cubital tunnel syndrome for surgical planning purposes. The presence of an anconeus epitrochlearis, ganglion cyst, and ulnohumeral osteophyte may cause or exacerbate cubital tunnel syndrome and can be detected by MR imaging (Fig. 3).

Additional pathologies may affect the ulnar nerve proximal and distal to the cubital tunnel. Snapping triceps syndrome is characterized by a snapping of the medial head of the triceps over the medial humeral epicondyle that may be asymptomatic, but can be associated with pain and ulnar neuritis.[39–41] It is an important entity to consider when evaluating the ulnar nerve at the elbow. The MR imaging may demonstrate ulnar neuritis proximal to the cubital tunnel and edema overlying the medial epicondyle. Dynamic ultrasonography is particularly useful in this clinical setting and should be considered for patients with ulnar neuritis at the elbow and associated snapping with movement.[41,42] Distal to the cubital tunnel masses can compress the nerve against the ulnar and humeral heads of the flexor carpi ulnaris (Fig. 4).

Guyon's canal
Guyon's canal is a potential site of ulnar nerve entrapment at the wrist. Patients present with variable sensory and/or motor symptoms depending on the location of entrapment and the branch involved.[43] Any space-occupying mass in Guyon's canal may result in symptoms. Causes of extrinsic compression of the ulnar nerve in Guyon's canal include ganglion cysts (Fig. 5), lipomas,[44] vascular lesions,[45–47] and accessory muscles.[48–51] Accessory muscles have been reported in up to 53% of wrists.[52] Guyon's canal syndrome may occur in the setting of repetitive (micro) trauma, and is classically associated with cyclists. In patients without clinically suspected Guyon's canal syndrome and an absence of anatomic abnormality, the T2-weighted signal of the nerve and secondary signs of intrinsic muscle denervation should be evaluated to determine if entrapment is present. Kollmer and colleagues[53] found T2-weighted hyperintensity of the deep branch of the ulnar nerve was higher in patients with Guyon's canal syndrome compared to asymptomatic volunteers.

RADIAL NERVE
Anatomy

C5, C6, C7, C8, and T1 contribute to the radial nerve via the posterior cord of the brachial plexus.

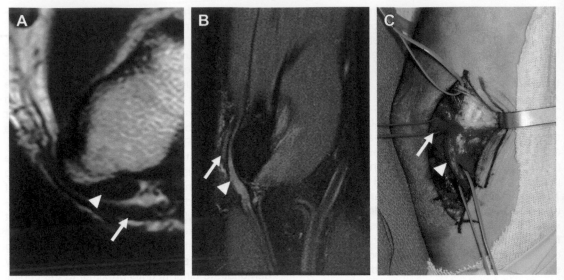

Fig. 3. Axial T1-weighted MR image the level of the cubital tunnel (*A*) demonstrates an anconeus epitrochlearis (*A, arrow*) adjacent to the ulnar nerve (*A, arrowhead*). A sagittal T2-weighted fat-saturated image through the cubital tunnel (*B*) also demonstrates the anconeus epitrochlearis (*B, arrow*). The nerve proximal to the cubital tunnel demonstrates enlargement and T2-weighted hyperintensity (*B, arrowhead*). The red vessel loop is around the accessory muscle (*C, arrow*) and the ulnar nerve is seen proximally (*C, arrowhead*).

The radial nerve crosses the lower axilla and passes deep to the proximal triceps muscles in the proximal arm. The radial nerve passes posterior to the proximal humerus in the spiral groove. It continues laterally in the lateral intermuscular septum of the arm deep to the brachioradialis muscle and travels anterior to the lateral humeral condyle. The bifurcation into the deep and superficial branches is located most commonly just distal to the radiocapitellar joint in the proximal forearm. The deep branch continues as the posterior interosseous nerve (PIN) after passing between the 2 heads of the supinator muscle. The

PIN arborizes at its exist from the supinator. The PIN lies along the posterior interosseous membrane of the forearm and terminates at the level of the extensor retinaculum of the wrist. The superficial branch of the radial nerve continues deep to the brachioradialis after the bifurcation. It travels adjacent to the radial artery in the proximal and mid forearm before passing deep to the brachioradialis tendon and extending superficially along the dorsum of the hand.

The radial nerve innervates the triceps brachii, anconeus, brachioradialis, and extensor carpi radialis longus above the elbow. The deep branch

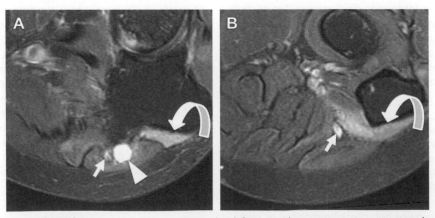

Fig. 4. Axial T2-weighted fat-saturated images at proximal forearm demonstrate an extraneural ganglion cyst arising from the ulnotrochlear margin of the joint (*A, arrowhead*). The cyst compresses the T2-weighted hyperintense and enlarged ulnar nerve (*A, B, arrows*) against the adjacent flexor carpi ulnaris. Denervation change is present in the proximal flexor digitorum profundus muscle (*A, B, curved arrows*).

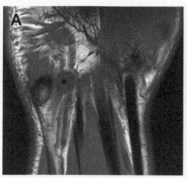
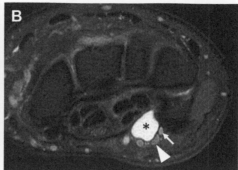

Fig. 5. Coronal T1-weighted (*A*) and axial T2-weighted fat-saturated (*B*) images of the wrist in a patient with ulnar neuropathy. A ganglion cyst (*A, B, asterisk*) is present in Guyon's canal. At the level of the pisiform (*B*) the cyst causes mass effect on the adjacent ulnar nerve. The deep (*B, arrow*) and superficial (*B, arrowhead*) branches are well seen and are displaced volar by the cyst. The deep branch (*B, arrow*) demonstrates increased T2-weighted signal compatible with neuritis.

of the radial nerve innervates the extensor carpi radialis brevis and supinator muscles and the PIN innervates the extensor compartment of the forearm (extensor digitorum, extensor digiti minimi, extensor carpi ulnaris, abductor pollicis longus, extensor pollicis brevis, extensor pollicis longus, and extensor indicis.) The radial nerve supplies sensation to a portion of the skin of the dorsal forearm. The superficial branch of the radial nerve provides sensation to the dorsum of the radial hand.

Pathology

Posterior interosseous nerve entrapment

Posterior interosseous neuropathy is also referred to as supinator syndrome. Compression of the PIN may lead to either motor weakness or a pain syndrome. PIN syndrome is notable posture of wrist dorsiflexion in a radial deviation and a finger drop (ie, loss of finger extension at the metacarpophangeal joints). The presence of pain is variable. A more controversial disorder known as radial tunnel syndrome is sometimes used in the setting of forearm pain without corresponding weakness thought to be owing to compression of the PIN.[54]

The deep branch of the radial nerve is susceptible to entrapment at a few different locations in the proximal forearm, the proximal edge of the supinator muscle (arcade of Froshe), the distal margin of the supinator muscle, the superomedial margin of the extensor carpi radialis brevis muscle, recurrent blood vessels (leash of Henry), and fibrous bands anterior to the joint.[55] Of the potential sites of entrapment, the proximal edge of the supinator

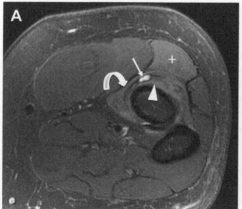
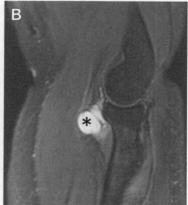

Fig. 6. Axial (*A*) and sagittal (*B*) T2-weighted fat-saturated images of the elbow in a patient with posterior interosseous neuropathy. The deep branch of the radial nerve demonstrates enlargement and T2-weighted hyperintensity (*A, arrow*) between the deep (*A, arrowhead*) and superficial (*A, curved arrow*) heads of the supinator muscle. Prominent radiobicipital bursitis (*B, asterisk*) is demonstrated compressing the nerve. Increased intramuscular T2-weighted signal is present in the supinator (*A, curved arrow* and *arrow head*) and extensor digitorum (*A, plus sign*) muscles, compatible with denervation.

at the arcade of Froshe is most often implicated.[55-57] The proximal margin of the supinator muscle varies in its membranous and fibrous composition, size, and thickness. A thick and fibrous arcade of Froshe may predispose to compression.[56] The arcade of Froshe is difficult to evaluate directly on MR imaging. MR diagnosis is typically made when a focal nerve enlargement and T2-weighted hyperintensity are identified at the proximal margin of the supinator muscle. MR imaging is also useful excluding PIN compression from a soft tissue mass (such as a lipoma), ganglion cyst, or an enlarged radiobicipital bursa (**Fig. 6**).

Superficial radial nerve

Isolated pathology of the superficial radial nerve is unusual. Referred to as Wartenberg syndrome, these patients present with pain over the dorsoradial aspect of the hand.[58] Dellon and Mackinnon[58] reported a series of 51 patients with superficial radial nerve entrapment and felt the entrapment occurred where the nerve passes through the fascia between the brachioradialis and the extensor carpi radialis longus tendons. MR imaging may demonstrate De Quervain disease, which is reported to be associated in 50% of cases[59] and may be helpful in excluding an extrinsic cause, such as a ganglion cyst.[60]

SUMMARY

Peripheral neuropathies are not uncommon and can be challenging for both those afflicted by them and for the clinicians tasked with the diagnosis and management of such disorders. Advances in cross-sectional imaging technologies and capabilities have aided considerably in the diagnosis of such disorders. When imaging studies remain inconclusive with regard to etiology, they may provide critical insight into lesion localization so as to aid in determining the safety or need for biopsy or resection of the causative lesion(s). Although ultrasonography has evolved greatly in recent years to aid in the diagnosis and evaluation of suspected peripheral neuropathies, particularly in cases where dynamic assessment is necessary, MR imaging has been and remains an invaluable tool in the evaluation of patients with suspected pathology of the peripheral nervous system. To reap the full benefit of the tremendous diagnostic capabilities of current imaging technology, a strong understanding of the anatomy and common sites of entrapment are imperative so as to facilitate proper protocol selection, adequate anatomic coverage, and ultimately accurate interpretation of the resultant findings.

REFERENCES

1. Chhabra A. Peripheral MR neurography: approach to interpretation. Neuroimaging Clin N Am 2014;24: 79–89.
2. Spinner RJ, Vincent JF, Wolanskyj AP, et al. Intraneural ganglion cyst: a 200-year-old mystery solved. Clin Anat 2008;21:611–8.
3. Zielinski CJ. Intraneural ganglion of the ulnar nerve at the wrist. Orthopedics 2003;26:429–30.
4. Spinner RJ, Wang H, Howe BM, et al. Deep ulnar intraneural ganglia in the palm. Acta Neurochir (Wien) 2012;154:1755–63.
5. Engstrom M, Thuomas KA, Naeser P, et al. Facial nerve enhancement in Bell's palsy demonstrated by different gadolinium-enhanced magnetic resonance imaging techniques. Arch Otolaryngol Head Neck Surg 1993;119:221–5.
6. Tien R, Dillon WP, Jackler RK. Contrast-enhanced MR imaging of the facial nerve in 11 patients with Bell's palsy. AJR Am J Roentgenol 1990;155:573–9.
7. Mauermann ML, Amrami KK, Kuntz NL, et al. Longitudinal study of intraneural perineurioma–a benign, focal hypertrophic neuropathy of youth. Brain 2009;132:2265–76.
8. Spinner RJ, Scheithauer BW, Amrami KK, et al. Adipose lesions of nerve: the need for a modified classification. J Neurosurg 2012;116:418–31.
9. Dailiana ZH, Bougioukli S, Varitimidis S, et al. Tumors and tumor-like lesions mimicking carpal tunnel syndrome. Arch Orthop Trauma Surg 2014;134:139–44.
10. Tahiri Y, Xu L, Kanevsky J, et al. Lipofibromatous hamartoma of the median nerve: a comprehensive review and systematic approach to evaluation, diagnosis, and treatment. J Hand Surg Am 2013; 38:2055–67.
11. Yalcinkaya M, Akman YE, Bagatur AE. Unilateral carpal tunnel syndrome caused by an occult ganglion in the carpal tunnel: a report of two cases. Case Rep Orthop 2014;2014:589021.
12. Yuen A, Thomson S. Carpal tunnel syndrome caused by heterotopic ossification. J Hand Surg Eur Vol 2011;36:425–6.
13. Hariri A, Cohen G, Masmejean EH. Venous malformation involving median nerve causing acute carpal tunnel syndrome. J Hand Surg Eur Vol 2011; 36:431–2.
14. Phalen GS. Reflections on 21 years' experience with the carpal-tunnel syndrome. JAMA 1970;212: 1365–7.
15. Phalen GS. The carpal-tunnel syndrome. Clinical evaluation of 598 hands. Clin Orthop Relat Res 1972;83:29–40.
16. Donato G, Galasso O, Valentino P, et al. Pathological findings in subsynovial connective tissue in idiopathic carpal tunnel syndrome. Clin Neuropathol 2009;28:129–35.

17. Jinrok O, Zhao C, Amadio PC, et al. Vascular pathologic changes in the flexor tenosynovium (subsynovial connective tissue) in idiopathic carpal tunnel syndrome. J Orthop Res 2004;22:1310–5.

18. Ettema AM, Zhao C, Amadio PC, et al. Gliding characteristics of flexor tendon and tenosynovium in carpal tunnel syndrome: a pilot study. Clin Anat 2007; 20:292–9.

19. Barcelo C, Faruch M, Lapegue F, et al. 3-T MRI with diffusion tensor imaging and tractography of the median nerve. Eur Radiol 2013;23:3124–30.

20. Cha JG, Han JK, Im SB, et al. Median nerve T2 assessment in the wrist joints: Preliminary study in patients with carpal tunnel syndrome and healthy volunteers. J Magn Reson Imaging 2014;40:789–95.

21. Lindberg PG, Feydy A, Le Viet D, et al. Diffusion tensor imaging of the median nerve in recurrent carpal tunnel syndrome - initial experience. Eur Radiol 2013;23:3115–23.

22. Naraghi A, da Gama Lobo L, Menezes R, et al. Diffusion tensor imaging of the median nerve before and after carpal tunnel release in patients with carpal tunnel syndrome: feasibility study. Skeletal Radiol 2013;42:1403–12.

23. Pham M, Baumer P, Meinck HM, et al. Anterior interosseous nerve syndrome: fascicular motor lesions of median nerve trunk. Neurology 2014;82:598–606.

24. Dunn AJ, Salonen DC, Anastakis DJ. MR imaging findings of anterior interosseous nerve lesions. Skeletal Radiol 2007;36:1155–62.

25. Gyftopoulos S, Rosenberg ZS, Petchprapa C. Increased MR signal intensity in the pronator quadratus muscle: Does it always indicate anterior interosseous neuropathy? AJR Am J Roentgenol 2010; 194:490–3.

26. Hartz CR, Linscheid RL, Gramse RR, et al. The pronator teres syndrome: compressive neuropathy of the median nerve. J Bone Joint Surg Am 1981;63: 885–90.

27. Seyffarth H. Primary myoses in the M. pronator teres as cause of lesion of the N. medianus (the pronator syndrome). Acta Psychiatr Neurol Scand Suppl 1951;74:251–4.

28. Tubbs RS, Marshall T, Loukas M, et al. The sublime bridge: anatomy and implications in median nerve entrapment. J Neurosurg 2010;113:110–2.

29. Andreisek G, Crook DW, Burg D, et al. Peripheral neuropathies of the median, radial, and ulnar nerves: MR imaging features. Radiographics 2006; 26:1267–87.

30. Gunnal SA, Siddiqui AU, Daimi SR, et al. A Study on the Accessory Head of the Flexor Pollicis Longus Muscle (Gantzer's Muscle). J Clin Diagn Res 2013; 7:418–21.

31. Natsis K. Supracondylar process of the humerus: study on 375 Caucasian subjects in Cologne, Germany. Clin Anat 2008;21:138–41.

32. Dellon AL. Musculotendinous variations about the medial humeral epicondyle. J Hand Surg 1986;11: 175–81.

33. Sookur PA, Naraghi AM, Bleakney RR, et al. Accessory muscles: anatomy, symptoms, and radiologic evaluation. Radiographics 2008;28:481–99.

34. Keen NN, Chin CT, Engstrom JW, et al. Diagnosing ulnar neuropathy at the elbow using magnetic resonance neurography. Skeletal Radiol 2012;41:401–7.

35. Baumer P, Dombert T, Staub F, et al. Ulnar neuropathy at the elbow: MR neurography–nerve T2 signal increase and caliber. Radiology 2011;260:199–206.

36. Britz GW, Haynor DR, Kuntz C, et al. Ulnar nerve entrapment at the elbow: correlation of magnetic resonance imaging, clinical, electrodiagnostic, and intraoperative findings. Neurosurgery 1996;38:458–65 [discussion: 465].

37. Vucic S, Cordato DJ, Yiannikas C, et al. Utility of magnetic resonance imaging in diagnosing ulnar neuropathy at the elbow. Clin Neurophysiol 2006; 117:590–5.

38. Husarik DB, Saupe N, Pfirrmann CW, et al. Elbow nerves: MR findings in 60 asymptomatic subjects–normal anatomy, variants, and pitfalls. Radiology 2009;252:148–56.

39. Spinner RJ, Goldner RD. Snapping of the medial head of the triceps: diagnosis and treatment. Tech Hand Up Extrem Surg 2002;6:91–7.

40. Spinner RJ, An KN, Kim KJ, et al. Medial or lateral dislocation (snapping) of a portion of the distal triceps: a biomechanical, anatomic explanation. J Shoulder Elbow Surg 2001;10:561–7.

41. Jacobson JA, Jebson PJ, Jeffers AW, et al. Ulnar nerve dislocation and snapping triceps syndrome: diagnosis with dynamic sonography–report of three cases. Radiology 2001;220:601–5.

42. Spinner RJ, Goldner RD, Lee RA. Diagnosis of snapping triceps with US. Radiology 2002;224:933–4 [author reply: 934].

43. Hoogvliet P, Coert JH, Friden J, et al. How to treat Guyon's canal syndrome? Results from the European HANDGUIDE study: a multidisciplinary treatment guideline. Br J Sports Med 2013;47:1063–70.

44. Ozdemir O, Calisaneller T, Gerilmez A, et al. Ulnar nerve entrapment in Guyon's canal due to a lipoma. J Neurosurg Sci 2010;54:125–7.

45. Dobson PF, Purushothaman B, Michla Y, et al. Delayed ulnar nerve palsy secondary to ulnar artery pseudoaneurysm distal to Guyon's canal following penetrating trauma to the hand. Ann R Coll Surg Engl 2013;95:e75–6.

46. Kim SS, Kim JH, Kang HI, et al. Ulnar Nerve Compression at Guyon's Canal by an Arteriovenous Malformation. J Korean Neurosurg Soc 2009;45:57–9.

47. Pai V, Harp A, Pai V. Guyon's canal syndrome: a rare case of venous malformation. J Hand Microsurg 2009;1:113–5.

48. Dimitriou C, Natsis K. Accessory abductor digiti minimi muscle causing ulnar nerve entrapment at the Guyon's canal: a case report. Clin Anat 2007;20: 974–5.

49. Harvie P, Patel N, Ostlere SJ. Ulnar nerve compression at Guyon's canal by an anomalous abductor digiti minimi muscle: the role of ultrasound in clinical diagnosis. Hand Surg 2003;8:271–5.

50. Paraskevas GK, Ioannidis O, Economou DS. Anomalous muscle causing ulnar nerve compression at Guyon's canal. J Plast Surg Hand Surg 2012;46: 288–90.

51. Spiess AM, Gursel E. Entrapment of the ulnar nerve at Guyon's canal by an accessory abductor digiti minimi muscle. Plast Reconstr Surg 2006;117: 1060–1.

52. Pierre-Jerome C, Moncayo V, Terk MR. The Guyon's canal in perspective: 3-T MRI assessment of the normal anatomy, the anatomical variations and the Guyon's canal syndrome. Surg Radiol Anat 2011; 33:897–903.

53. Kollmer J, Baumer P, Milford D, et al. T2-signal of ulnar nerve branches at the wrist in Guyon's canal syndrome. PLoS One 2012;7:e47295.

54. Naam NH, Nemani S. Radial tunnel syndrome. Orthop Clin North Am 2012;43:529–36.

55. Konjengbam M, Elangbam J. Radial nerve in the radial tunnel: anatomic sites of entrapment neuropathy. Clin Anat 2004;17:21–5.

56. Spinner M. The arcade of Frohse and its relationship to posterior interosseous nerve paralysis. J Bone Joint Surg Br 1968;50:809–12.

57. Thomas SJ, Yakin DE, Parry BR, et al. The anatomical relationship between the posterior interosseous nerve and the supinator muscle. J Hand Surg Am 2000;25:936–41.

58. Dellon AL, Mackinnon SE. Radial sensory nerve entrapment. Arch Neurol 1986;43:833–5.

59. Lanzetta M, Foucher G. Entrapment of the superficial branch of the radial nerve (Wartenberg's syndrome). A report of 52 cases. Int Orthop 1993;17: 342–5.

60. Sirrajelhak M, Fnini S, Arssi M, et al. Compression of the superficial branch of the radial nerve by a synovial ganglion of the elbow (about one case and literature review). Chir Main 2013;32:255–7 [in French].

Magnetic Resonance Angiography of the Upper Extremity

Peter Bannas, MD[a,b,*], Christopher J. François, MD[a],
Scott B. Reeder, MD, PhD[a,c,d,e,f]

KEYWORDS

- Magnetic resonance imaging • MR angiography • MRA • Contrast-enhanced MRA
- Upper extremity • Peripheral arteries

KEY POINTS

- Magnetic resonance angiography (MRA) can provide excellent image quality with high spatial resolution of the vessels of the upper extremity.
- Time-resolved MRA can be used to depict the flow dynamics of pathology to the upper extremity in the same way that digital subtraction angiography (DSA) provides functional information about vascular pathology.
- Practicing radiologists should be familiar with MRA imaging techniques used for individual cases to establish a correct diagnosis.
- MRA techniques must to be tailored for each individual to achieve optimal image quality and maximal diagnostic yield.
- Contrast-enhanced MRA (CE-MRA) techniques are currently preferred to noncontrast MRA techniques for imaging the upper extremity.

INTRODUCTION

MRA is a noninvasive imaging modality with high spatial resolution that can be used for diagnosis and treatment planning of vascular abnormalities of the upper extremity.[1,2] Unlike CT angiography (CTA) or DSA, it avoids the need for ionizing radiation and exposure to iodinated contrast agents. Targeted MRA of anatomic regions, such as the hand, can achieve high spatial resolution and in some instances may surpass the performance of CTA. In addition, the high attenuation of bone necessitates the need for complex postprocessing algorithms that segment bone from CTAs, because bone can obscure the visualization of small arteries of the distal extremities. DSA has the highest spatial and temporal resolution and remains the standard of reference for imaging the upper extremity. Recent developments in MRA, however, including time-resolved imaging, have made dynamic imaging of the vasculature feasible in the clinical setting to assess the anatomic and hemodynamic abnormalities seen in vascular disease and to bring MRA closer to the DSA reference standard.[1]

The Authors have nothing to disclose.
[a] Department of Radiology, University of Wisconsin-Madison, 600 Highland Avenue, Madison, WI 53792-3252, USA; [b] Department of Radiology, University Hospital Hamburg-Eppendorf, Martinistrasse 52, Hamburg 20246, Germany; [c] Department of Biomedical Engineering, University of Wisconsin-Madison, 1415 Engineering Drive, Madison, WI 53706, USA; [d] Department of Medical Physics, University of Wisconsin-Madison, 1111 Highland Avenue, Madison, WI 53705-2275, USA; [e] Department of Medicine, University of Wisconsin-Madison, 1685 Highland Avenue, Madison, WI 53705-2281, USA; [f] Department of Emergency Medicine, University of Wisconsin-Madison, 600 Highland Avenue, Madison, WI 53792, USA
* Corresponding author. Department of Radiology, University of Wisconsin-Madison, 600 Highland Avenue, Room E1/372, Madison, WI 53792-3252.
E-mail address: p.bannas@uke.de

Magn Reson Imaging Clin N Am 23 (2015) 479–493
http://dx.doi.org/10.1016/j.mric.2015.04.004
1064-9689/15/$ – see front matter © 2015 Elsevier Inc. All rights reserved.

MRA of the upper extremity can be performed with or without the use of contrast agents. Although CE-MRA is generally preferred, non–contrast-enhanced techniques are increasingly available and may be a good option for patients with impaired renal function or who have allergies to gadolinium-based contrast agents (GBCAs). Non–contrast-enhanced techniques often overestimate stenoses in the setting of complex vessel anatomy or abnormal blood flow and can be time consuming. CE-MRA is robust and less time consuming. A major challenge for all CE-MRA techniques is to achieve optimal timing of the contrast bolus relative to the sampling of the center of k-space, which is crucial for optimal imaging. The specific MRA protocol chosen should be tailored to the patient to provide the best possible image quality.

A broad spectrum of vascular disorders of the upper extremity, ranging from the thoracic outlet syndrome to distal disease, such as thromboangiitis obliterans and hypothenar hammer syndrome, can be assessed accurately using MRA of the upper extremity. This review discusses MRA techniques and MRA findings of common disease entities of the upper extremity.

MRA TECHNIQUES

The main requisite for diagnostic MRA is to achieve sufficient spatial resolution and sufficient vessel contrast.[3] A high-field magnetic resonance (MR) scanner (1.5T or 3T) with modern phased-array receive coils is necessary to obtain images with high spatial resolution and high signal-to-noise ratio, while still covering the region of interest. Dedicated phased-array extremity or wrist coils should be used whenever possible, depending on the region of interest and required coverage.

Contrast-Enhanced MRA Techniques

Contrast-enhanced MRA
Of all available methods, CE-MRA has evolved as the preferred technique for MR imaging of the arterial vasculature.[3] CE-MRA relies on the T1 shortening effect of paramagnetic GBCAs. This results in a significant difference in signal intensity between blood and adjacent tissue when using heavily T1-weighted arterial-phase imaging.[3] The image acquisition must be timed with the contrast bolus peak during the sampling of the center of k-space to achieve maximum vessel contrast. Before the contrast material is injected, a nonenhanced acquisition with the same sequence settings as the contrast-enhanced scans can be acquired to allow for subtraction with the subsequent arterial-phase images. Subtracted images can be further manipulated with a maximum intensity projection (MIP) visualization to produce 3-D representations of the arterial anatomy.[2] Recent approaches in the lower extremity using Dixon-based methods are an alternative approach that can be used to suppress background fat signal potentially obviating subtraction.[4] This approach is promising for lower extremity MRA and also may be helpful for MRA of the upper extremity.

The advantages of CE-MRA include short scan times and high spatial resolution with minimal flow-related artifacts.[2] CE-MRA findings are highly reproducible, and image quality is comparable to that of DSA.[5] The main disadvantage of CE-MRA is the need for injection of GBCA, which has been associated with nephrogenic systemic fibrosis (NSF) in patients with renal insufficiency.[6] Overall, however, the safety profile of GBCAs is excellent and generally exceeds that of iodinated agents.[7]

Time-resolved MRA
Temporal resolution can add clinically valuable information to an examination of the upper extremity, including collateral flow pathways associated with stenoses and visualization of arterial to venous shunting. Another major advantage of time-resolved imaging is that it obviates a timing bolus or real-time fluorotriggering techniques. In this way, time-resolved imaging provides a point-and-shoot approach that is highly advantageous for imaging challenging anatomy where bolus timing/triggering methods are impractical.[8]

Most time-resolved MRA techniques use view-sharing methods to achieve high temporal resolution while maintaining high spatial resolution.[9] Such approaches use frequent sampling of low spatial frequencies (center of k-space) with less frequent sampling of higher spatial frequencies (periphery of k-space) that are subsequently shared between the final reconstructed 3-D data sets. These methods are commonly used in combination with subtraction, obtained by acquiring a precontrast mask, ultimately providing a set of time-resolved 3-D data images showing progressive enhancement of vessels akin to DSA. A major advantage is that not only morphologic but also dynamic information is obtained, which may allow for evaluation of the hemodynamic relevance of a stenosis. From the rapidly acquired multiple images, the best arterial or other relevant phase can be chosen. Time-resolved MRA can be performed in the same imaging session together with high-resolution standard MRA for more detailed depiction of small vessels.

Noncontrast MRA

Time of flight (TOF) and phase contrast (PC) are currently the most commonly used noncontrast MRA techniques.[10] Newer techniques are ECG-gated balanced steady-state free precession, flow-sensitive dephasing, and arterial spin labeling techniques.[11] Appropriate use of these techniques can allow diagnosis of vascular diseases in patients with chronic kidney disease without using contrast materials.[12]

Time of flight MRA

TOF MRA is based on the principle that the protons in blood flowing into a presaturated imaging section of interest are unsaturated and thereby provide fresh magnetization when excited with the radiofrequency pulse.[11] A major advantage of TOF MRA is that no contrast agents are required. Furthermore, by placing a saturation band above or below the section of interest, the direction of blood flow can be assessed. Disadvantages of this method include small imaging volumes, long acquisition times, and artifacts related to either slow or turbulent flow. These artifacts can impede assessment of vascular disease, potentially causing false-positive overdetection of vascular stenoses.[3]

Phase-contrast MRA

PC MRA requires the acquisition of 2 or more (typically 4) data sets[13] or flow-compensated pulses to generate flow-sensitive phase images. Phase data can be used either to reconstruct velocity-encoded flow-quantification images or MRA images.[14] This technique is commonly used for flow imaging and measurement of flow but only in rare cases is it used for pure angiographic imaging of the upper extremity. The direction of flow can also be depicted with PC imaging and may be helpful verifying the presence of functionally significant vascular pathology.

IMAGING PROTOCOL
Contrast Agents

CE-MRA can be performed with any extracellular contrast agents, such as gadopentetate dimeglumine (Magnevist, Bayer HealthCare, Whippany, New Jersey).[15,16] Furthermore, there has been great interest in the use of high relaxivity agents, such as gadobenate dimeglumine (MultiHance, Bracco Diagnostics, Princeton, New Jersey)[17,18] or gadobutrol (Bayer HealthCare, Wayne, New Jersey).[19] Extracellular contrast agents have a short blood pool half-life and are best suited for arterial-phase or early delayed-phase imaging. This makes the need for accurate bolus timing important.

The limitations of imaging with extracellular agents led to the development of intravascular contrast agents with a prolonged intravascular half-life, referred to as blood pool contrast agents. Gadofosveset trisodium (Lantheus Medical Imaging, North Billerica, Massachusetts) binds reversibly to human serum albumin, which effectively prolongs the serum half-life to several hours.[20] As with other extracellular contrast agents, first-pass MRA can be performed with gadofosveset. The main advantage of gadofosveset is the ability to perform steady state imaging that is helpful for facilitating delayed imaging using provocative maneuvers, such as arm position, to evaluate for thoracic outlet syndrome.

Injection Protocol

The contrast agent should be injected at a minimum rate of 1.5 to 2 mL/s using a power injector followed by a 30- to 50-mL saline flush at the same rate. Injecting the contrast agent in the contralateral extremity (from that with suspected pathology) avoids susceptibility artifacts due to high concentrations of gadolinium during first pass of the injection in the symptomatic extremity (Fig. 1).[21] In some circumstances, it may be necessary to inject from a foot vein or femoral central venous access. Furthermore, dilution of contrast agents in saline to large bolus volumes (approximately 30 mL) is an off-label practice that the authors find helpful for prolonging the contrast bolus and providing better matching of a uniform bolus during the k-space acquisition. Dilution of contrast may also be helpful when small volumes of contrast (eg, with an infant or small child) are needed and are difficult to handle using power injectors. Dilution also mitigate susceptibility related artifacts from highly concentrated contrast.

Positioning of the Patient

Patient comfort is of paramount importance to ensure a successful examination with minimal motion artifact. Feet-first imaging may be recommended for claustrophobic patients, but head-first imaging allows the injection site to be monitored and is preferable. For upper arm imaging, patients should be positioned supine with the arm next to the body. The arm and site of interest should be moved as close as possible to the center of the magnet. For forearm and hand imaging, patients should be positioned in a decubitus prone position, with the arm of interest extended above the head (superman position). The arm and region of interest should be positioned within the extremity coil as close to the center of the magnet as

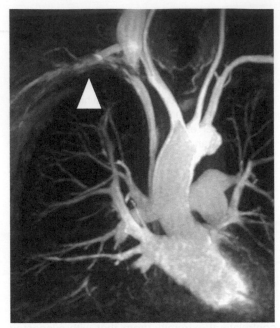

Fig. 1. Susceptibility artifact. The high concentration of gadolinium during first pass of the injection leads to a susceptibility artifact with signal drop in the right subclavian vein as well as in the adjacent subclavian artery (*arrowhead*). Injecting the contrast agent in the contralateral extremity (from that with suspected pathology) avoids susceptibility artifacts in the symptomatic extremity. Dilution also mitigates susceptibility related artifacts from highly concentrated contrast.

possible. In cases of clinically suspected vasospasm, wrapping the hand in a warm towel may be helpful in depicting the peripheral digital vessels.[2] When the hand is imaged, the palm should lie flat within the coil with the fingers slightly spread to include the entire arterial tree in the imaging volume.[2]

MRA Protocols

Proximal upper extremity

Imaging of the proximal upper extremity should be performed with phased-array receive coils. The authors use an 8-element cardiac coil that is placed over a patient's chest and arm of interest. In general, a single-phase MRA can be performed for imaging of the proximal upper extremity; however, time-resolved MRA can also be performed to assess the flow dynamics. The single PC-enhanced MRA can be performed coronal or coronal-oblique. The authors use a 3-D spoiled gradient-echo sequence with a repetition time (TR) of 3.0 to 3.5 ms and an echo time (TE) of 1.0 to 1.2 ms, 25 to 30 flip angle, field of view (FOV) approximately 30 38 cm, approximately 192 256 matrix, and 1.6- to 2.0-mm slice thickness. Zero-filling in the in-plane

and through plane direction is recommended to avoid stair-step artifacts when performing multiplanar reformatting (MPR).

Forearm

Imaging of the forearm should be performed with dedicated phased-array extremity coils. The authors use either an 8-element cardiac coil or 16-element extremity wrap coils. In general, a time-resolved MRA should be performed for imaging of the forearm. The authors recommend performing the excitation in sagittal orientation to avoid foldover (wrapping) artifacts from the body. The authors use 3-D time-resolved imaging of contrast kinetics (TRICKS)[9] with a TR of 3.5 to 4.0 ms and a TE of 1.0 to 1.4 ms, 25 to 30 flip angle, FOV approximately 13 42 cm, approximately 320 320 matrix, and 1.6- to 2.0-mm slice thickness. Zero-filling is performed to facilitate interpolation, necessary to performing MPRs.

Hand

Imaging of the hand should be performed with dedicated phased-array extremity coils. The authors use a 16-element extremity wrap coil or a quadrature knee coil. In general, a time-resolved MRA should always be performed for imaging of the hand. We use 3-D TRICKS[9] with a TR of 2.8 to 3.0 ms and a TE of 1.0–1.2 ms, 25 to 30 flip angle, FOV approximately 14.4 24 cm, approximately 224 256 matrix, and 1.2- to 1.8-mm slice thickness. Zero-filling is performed to facilitate interpolation, necessary to perform MPRs.

CLINICAL APPLICATIONS
Subclavian Steal Syndrome

The subclavian steal syndrome is caused by a stenosis or occlusion of the proximal subclavian artery or the brachiocephalic trunk.[22] The stenosis/occlusion leads to retrograde blood flow in the vertebral artery to supply the affected arm with blood at the expense of the vertebrobasilar circulation, hence the name subclavian steal.[23] This steal may cause symptoms, such as vertigo, presyncope, syncope, and even stroke, and is often exacerbated by exercise of the affected upper extremity. Atherosclerosis is the most common cause of subclavian stenosis, although any pathology, such as vasculitis, that affects the arch vessels can lead to this syndrome. The prevalence is less than 2% in the general population and a majority of cases are asymptomatic.[24]

MRA not only can assess the severity of the stenosis/occlusion but also can demonstrate the presence of reversed flow in the vertebral artery.[25] CE-MRA should be used to localize and quantify the degree of the stenosis of the proximal subclavian artery (**Fig. 2**). TOF MRA with appropriate saturation bands, time-resolved CE-MRA, and PC MRA all can demonstrate retrograde flow in the vertebral artery (see **Fig. 2**). In the authors' experience, PC imaging in a single axial plane with flow encoding in the superior/inferior direction is a rapid and unambiguous method to demonstrate flow reversal in a vertebral artery.

Takayasu Arteritis

Takayasu arteritis is an uncommon form of large-vessel granulomatous vasculitis.[26] The inflammatory process results in stenosis, occlusion, dilatation, or aneurysm formation in the arterial wall. It affects mainly the aorta and its branches but may also affect other vessels, such as the pulmonary arteries. The left subclavian artery may be involved in up to 50% of patients.[27] Patients develop systemic symptoms during an initial inflammatory phase, such as malaise, fever, night sweats, weight loss, arthralgia, and fatigue. Patients may also develop anemia and elevated C-reactive protein, although these are not reliable for diagnosis. The initial phase is often followed by a secondary pulseless phase, characterized by vascular stenoses and occlusions from intimal narrowing. The disease is more frequently in the Asian population and in young women (<50 years of age).

MRA aids in diagnosis and allows for assessment of the extent of disease.[28] CE-MRA allows detection of typical findings, such as luminal narrowing from arterial stenosis, occlusion, or dilatation (**Fig. 3**). Fat-suppressed T2-weighted imaging is helpful to assess vessel wall edema and perivascular inflammation, particularly in the early, active stages. Postcontrast T1-weighted fat-saturated imaging shows thickening and enhancement of the vessel walls in patients with active disease.

Giant Cell Arteritis

Giant cell arteritis (GCA), also known as temporal arteritis or Horton disease, is the most common chronic vasculitis of medium- and large-sized arteries in persons ages 50 and older.[29] The characteristic histopathologic features of GCA include granulomatous inflammation of the vessel wall with multinucleated giant cells.[30] The involvement of epicranial arteries facilitates histopathologic

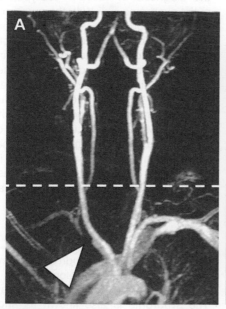
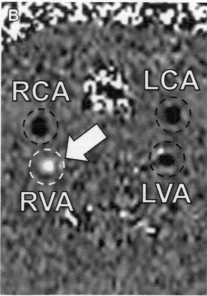

Fig. 2. Subclavian steal syndrome. (*A*) Coronal MIP image of a contrast-enhanced 3-D time-resolved MRA demonstrates short segment occlusion (*arrowhead*) at the origin of the right proximal subclavian artery. The occlusion is located just distal to the origin of the right common carotid artery but proximal of the origin of the right vertebral artery. Note the delayed enhancement of the right subclavian artery compared with the fully enhanced left subclavian artery. Contrast agent was injected from the left arm to avoid first-pass venous overlay of the area of interest on the affected right side. (*B*) Axial PC image demonstrates reversal (caudad) of flow in the right vertebral artery (RVA) (*white, arrow*) compared with cephalad flow in the left vertebral artery (LVA) (*black*) and common carotid arteries, right carotid artery (RCA) and left carotid artery (LCA) (*black*). The dotted line (*A*) indicates the level of the axial PC section (*B*).

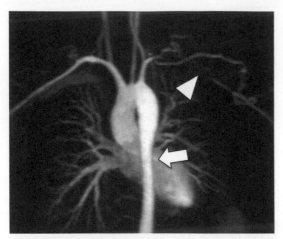

Fig. 3. Takaysu arteritis in a 34-year-old woman. Coronal MIP of contrast-enhanced 3-D time-resolved MRA demonstrates a long-segment complete occlusion (*arrowhead*) of the left subclavian artery with supply of the distal artery via a collateral vessel. Also the descending aorta has a tapered narrowing (*arrow*). The other vessels are of normal caliber without occlusion or stenosis. Although this is an example of complete occlusion, long-segment stenosis is also common in Takayasu arteritis. Contrast was injected from the nonaffected right arm to avoid first-pass venous overlay of the symptomatic side.

confirmation. The superficial temporal artery, however, may not be involved, and establishing a diagnosis of GCA may be challenging if other vessels, such as the subclavian arteries, are affected.

MRA is helpful for diagnosis and assessment of disease extent in GCA.[31] MRA can identify the localization and inflammatory changes of the arteries and guides clinicians to alternative biopsy sites when initial results are negative.[1,32] MRA findings include segmental smooth arterial stenoses alternating with normal-caliber or dilated segments.[1] The stenoses are smooth and tapered (**Fig. 4**). Extraluminal findings may include wall thickening, hyperintensity in the vessel wall on fat-suppressed T2-weighted images, and wall

enhancement on delayed-phase imaging.[32,33] In general, the findings of GCA are often indistinguishable from Takayasu arteritis. Patient age, presentation, and other clinical information, including biopsy and/or laboratory values, may be needed to distinguish the 2 entities. Distinguishing these 2 types of arteritis based on clinical information is usually straightforward.

Thoracic Outlet Syndrome

The thoracic outlet syndrome is caused by a compression of the brachial plexus or subclavian vessels as they pass between the chest and upper extremity (thoracic outlet) between the anterior and middle scalene muscles.[34] The syndrome may be positional due to abnormal compression from the clavicle when the arm is elevated. There are also several static forms, including aberrant positioning of the first rib, presence of a cervical rib, and hypertrophy of scalene muscles from athletic training (eg, with baseball pitchers). In cases of vascular thoracic outlet syndrome, symptoms may include discoloration of the affected arm, weakness of the arm muscles, and tingling.

MRA with positional maneuvers, such as superior positioning of the arm, is particularly useful in the diagnosis of vascular subtypes of thoracic outlet syndrome.[35,36] With the arm(s) up, localization of stenotic lesions during provocative arm positioning is helpful for differentiation between positional and static causes (**Fig. 5**). First, a coronal oblique arterial and venous-phase CE-MRA should be acquired during greater than or equal to 150 to 160 of bilateral arm abduction with the head and neck in the neutral position. Time-resolved MRA is particularly useful during this phase. The arms are then repositioned next to the torso, and delayed venous-phase images are obtained.[35] If an intravascular contrast agent is used, a second injection during the arms-down phase is not necessary.

Paget-Schroetter Syndrome

The Paget-Schroetter syndrome is a rare condition that describes the development of deep vein thrombosis of the axillary and subclavian veins. The syndrome is also known as effort-induced thrombosis because is it is often associated with exertion and mechanical stress, but it can also occur spontaneously or secondary to other causes.[37] The increased use of central venous catheters has been associated with an increasing rate of upper extremity thrombosis.[38] Symptoms include sudden onset of pain, warmth, redness, blueness, and swelling of the upper extremity.

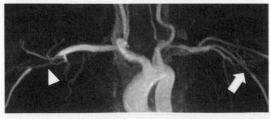

Fig. 4. GCA in a 71-year-old woman. Coronal MIP of contrast-enhanced 3-D time-resolved MRA demonstrates a long-segment high-grade stenosis of the right subclavian artery (*arrowhead*) and a long-segment moderate stenosis of the left subclavian artery (*arrow*).

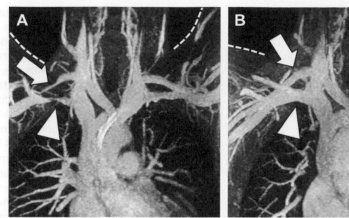

Fig. 5. Thoracic outlet syndrome in a patient with small bilateral cervical ribs. Coronal MIP of contrast-enhanced 3-D MRA with (*A*) elevated and (*B*) lowered arms demonstrating a positional cause of thoracic outlet syndrome. With the arms positioned above the head, there is severe external compression of the right subclavian artery (*arrows*) and vein (*arrowheads*) between the clavicle and the rib cage. There is also a mild compression of the left subclavian vein. The compression resolves when the arms are down. Note that this examination has been performed with an intravascular contrast agent, gadofosveset trisodium, with a long intravascular half-life. This enabled repeated imaging with dynamic positioning of the arms using a single-contrast injection. Dotted lines indicate the position of the arms. The cervical rib on the rights side was resected after the diagnosis.

MRA can be used to confirm the presence and the extent of thrombosis and to assess underlying reasons, such as osseous or muscular abnormalities and the presence of inflammation (**Fig. 6**). Contrast-enhanced MR venography allows visualization not only of the axillary and subclavian veins but also of the central veins of the thorax with high sensitivity and specificity.[39] MRA also offers the opportunity to assess the presence of pulmonary embolism within the same imaging session.[18,40] Contrast-enhanced MR venography can be performed indirectly, via injection of the GBCA in the contralateral extremity and subsequent repeated delayed-phase imaging or time-resolved MRA, or, alternatively, direct MR venography can be performed by slow injection of dilute contrast in the

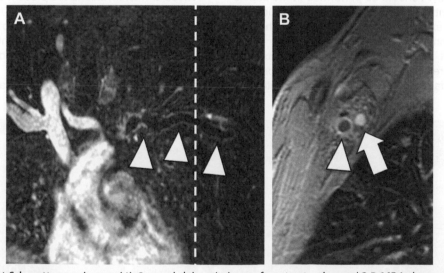

Fig. 6. Paget-Schroetter syndrome. (*A*) Coronal delayed-phase of contrast-enhanced 3-D MRA demonstrates low signal intensity within the lumen of the left subclavian vein consistent with thrombus (*arrowheads*). Note that the contrast agent was injected via a lower extremity to avoid any first-pass venous overlay of both upper extremities. (*B*) Sagittal postcontrast T1-weighted images confirm the complete thrombotic occlusion of the left subclavian vein (*arrowhead*) next to the patent subclavian artery (*arrow*). Note the enhancement of the vessel of wall of the vein. The dotted line (*A*) indicates the level of the section (*B*).

affected extremity upstream of the thrombosis typically in a dorsal hand vein.[41] Ruehm and colleagues[41] recommended a dilution of 1:15 using gadopentetate dimeglumine, although agents with higher transverse relaxivity, such as gadobenate dimeglumine,[42] may require more dilution to avoid deleterious effects of T2* decay at high-contrast concentrations.

Arteriovenous Fistulas for Hemodialysis

The arteriovenous fistula (AVF) is commonly used for hemodialysis vascular access. The AVF is created surgically and shunts blood from the artery to the vein by end-to-side anastomosis of the radial or brachial artery to the adjacent vein.[43] Unfortunately, access complications, such as thrombosis and stenosis, are common and require early recognition and treatment to avoid failure of the fistula, necessitating creation of a new AVF.[44] Stenosis can occur anywhere along the arteriovenous circuit, and diagnostic imaging of the entire graft is necessary. Furthermore, the high flow state can lead to central vessel stenosis, and visualization of the vasculature of the entire extremity proximal to the AVF up to the arch and superior vena cava is required when evaluating the AVF.[1]

MRA allows noninvasive detection and monitoring of hemodynamic stenosis with the advantage of imaging over a large FOV.[45] Time-resolved MRA permits noninvasive dynamic monitoring of the filling of the arterial and venous vessels.[46,47] Coronal or oblique coronal time-resolved MRA should be performed in the supine position with the arms at the side of the body to cover the extremity of interest to include the AVF and the contiguous chest (Fig. 7).

Contrast agents (both iodinated agents and GCBAs) are generally contraindicated in patients with renal failure due to the potential nephrotoxicity of iodinated agents or the potential risk of NSF from GBCAs. In general, the authors believe the risk of NSF is low and can be mitigated using group II agents and with low doses although not entirely eliminated. Because these patients are, by definition, dialysis dependent, care should be taken to coordinate MRA with dialysis. Although dialysis may not protect patients who are exposed to GBCAs from developing NSF,[48] it is generally recommended that dialysis be performed within 24 hours after gadolinium administration.[49] Furthermore, the lowest dose possible should be used and the use of group II agents (ie, those agents with few, if any, unconfounded cases of NSF) are generally suggested in circumstances where the potential (but low) risk of NSF is outweighed by the need to obtain important diagnostic information.[50] Group II GBCAs include gadobenate dimeglumine (MultiHance), gadoteridol (ProHance, Bracco Diagnostics), gadoteric acid (Dotarem, Guerbet, Roissy CdG, France), and gadobutrol (Gadavist).[50]

Vascular Anomalies

Vascular manifestations of various disease entities may involve the upper extremity.[51] Hemangioma is a well-defined entity that should be differentiated from the general class of vascular malformations.[52] Hemangioma is an endothelial hyperplasia consisting of lobules of microcapillaries. It may be absent or small at birth and grows rapidly with 2 successive phases of proliferation and regression.

Vascular malformations are present at birth and do not exhibit endothelial anomalies. Their growth parallels that of the child and they do not regress.[53] Vascular malformations are classified into low-flow (venous, lymphatic, and capillary) and high-flow (arteriovenous lesions and fistulae) malformations.[52] MRA in combination with standard MR

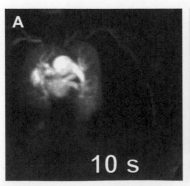
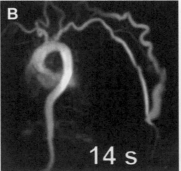
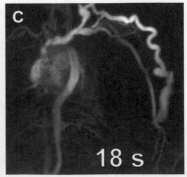

Fig. 7. AVF for hemodialysis. Time-resolved MRA permits noninvasive dynamic monitoring of the filling of the arterial and venous vessels. (A–C) Three time frames of coronal MIPs of contrast-enhanced 3-D time-resolved MRA demonstrate patency of the AVF and allow for exclusion of thrombi. (*Courtesy of* James Carr, MD, Departments of Radiology and Biomedical Engineering, Northwestern University, Chicago, IL.)

imaging sequences, such as T2-weighted imaging, can help differentiate these entities.[51]

Hemangioma

As discussed previously, the term, *hemangioma*, should be reserved for true vascular tumors.[51,52] *Infantile hemangioma* should be strictly reserved for a lesion occurring in a child. Pediatric cutaneous vascular lesions and hemangiomas are often absent or small at birth and grow rapidly with 2 successive phases of proliferation, followed by near or complete regression, typically by the age of 7.[51] Therefore, it is uncommon for adolescents or adults to have a true hemangioma.[54]

Intramuscular hemangioma is a rare and distinct entity that affects striated muscle and is typically found in adolescents or young adults. As opposed to infantile hemangioma, it appears rapidly and never regresses.[51] It is formed not only by abnormal vessels but also by a soft tissue mass unlike other vascular malformations. Nonvascular elements, such as fat, muscle, bone, fibrous tissue, hemosiderin, and thrombus, may be present.[55] The intramuscular hemangioma is characterized by rapid growth and usually only affects a single muscle.

MRA, together with standard MR imaging sequences, allows for assessment of size, extent, and feeding and draining vessels. The soft tissue mass is typically hyperintense signal on T2-weighted imaging and intermediate intensity on T1-weighted imaging. Flow voids may be present due to high-flow vessels. Coronal (time-resolved) MRA or MR imaging shows strong enhancement of the soft tissue mass due to hypervascularization formed by arteries and arterioles, but there is no early venous drainage as seen with arteriovenous malformations (AVMs) (**Fig. 8**). Within the soft tissue mass there might be areas with reduced enhancement due to the presence of nonvascular components, such as fat, fibrous tissue, calcification, or thrombus.[51] Confident differentiation of hemangioma from true vascular malformation may be difficult, although the presence of a soft tissue mass is the most reliable sign of a hemangioma (**Fig. 9**).[51]

Venous malformations

Venous malformations are the most frequently encountered type of vascular malformation. They are found usually in children or young adults. Symptoms include localized pain, soft tissue

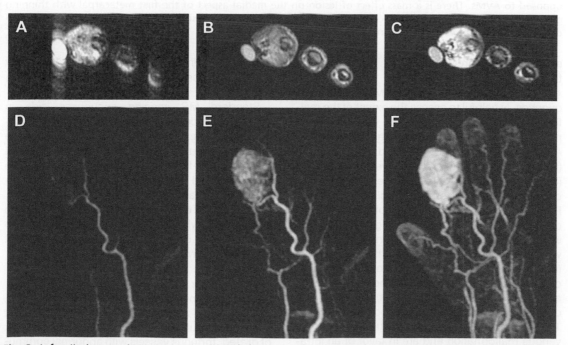

Fig. 8. Infantile hemangioma in 2-year-old girl. (*A*) Axial fat-suppressed T2-weighted imaging demonstrates a hyperintense soft tissue mass along the radial aspect of the second digit. (*B*) The mass has intermediate signal intensity on precontrast T1-weighted images. (*C*) Axial postcontrast T1-weighted images in the delayed arterial phase demonstrate strong enhancement of the mass but no early drainage as opposed to AVMs. (*D–F*) Three time frames of coronal MIPs of contrast-enhanced 3-D time-resolved MRA demonstrate enhancement of the soft tissue mass that follows the enhancement of the arteries.

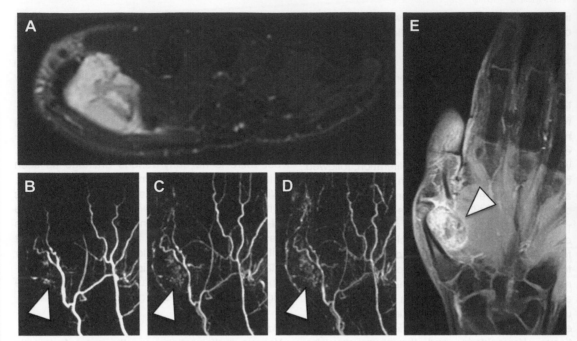

Fig. 9. Intramuscular hemangioma in a 40-year-old woman. (*A*) Axial fat-suppressed T2-weighted imaging demonstrates a hyperintense soft tissue mass along the medial aspect of the first metacarpal. The mass has hypointense punctate internal areas corresponding to calcifications seen on conventional radiographs (not shown). (*B–D*) Three time frames of coronal MIPs of contrast-enhanced 3-D time-resolved MRA demonstrate enhancement of the soft tissue mass (*arrowheads*) that follows the enhancement of the arteries. (*E*) Coronal postcontrast T1-weighted images demonstrate strong enhancement of the mass (*arrowhead*) but no early drainage as opposed to AVMs. There is a mass effect of lesion on the medial aspect of the first metacarpal with thinning of the metacarpal itself. The presence of soft tissue mass is most reliable sign of a hemangioma for differential diagnosis with other vascular malformations.

swelling, and, rarely, decreased functionality of the involved extremity.

MRA, together with standard MR imaging sequences, is helpful to assess the extent of the malformation and the relationship of the venous malformation with feeding and draining vessels.[51] Axial fat-suppressed T2-weighted fast spin-echo (FSE) imaging or short tau inversion recovery (STIR) FSE shows high signal due the high water content in the venous blood pools of the lesion. Phleboliths may be present as punctuate signal dropouts on T1- and T2-weighted imaging, whereas areas of high signal intensity on T1-weighted images may represent thrombi. Coronal (time-resolved) MRA shows a prominent nodular or tubular enhancement of the venous blood pools and depicts the relationship to the feeding and draining vessels.[51] Flow voids both on T1- and T2-weighted spin-echo techniques rule out a venous malformation and are in favor of an intramuscular hemangioma or AVM.[51]

Lymphatic malformations

Lymphatic malformations are seen more frequently in the cephalic, axillary, and thoracic regions than in the upper extremity. They may suddenly increase in size and become painful to palpation.[51]

Standard MR imaging sequences aids in diagnosis by identifying fluid-filled micro- or macrocystic cysts. The cysts have low signal on T1-weighted and high signal on T2-weighted images. Fluid-fluid levels may be present, due to intralesional bleeding or accumulation of proteinaceous material. During dynamic CE-MRA, enhancement of the walls and septae can be appreciated, whereas the content of the cysts do not enhance, unlike venous malformations that demonstrate avid enhancement.[51]

Arteriovenous malformations

AVMs are typically characterized by a warm, reddish mass and may feature a systolic bruit heard at auscultation. AVMs consist of a network of dilated, tortuous vessels with abnormal communications between arteries and veins that infiltrate and often replace surrounding normal tissue.[53]

MRA, together with standard MR imaging sequences, allows further characterization and delineation of the feeding and draining vessels.[51]

Both, T1- and T2-weighted sequences show numerous tubular structures that have multiple signal (flow) voids (spin-echo techniques) due to high arterial or arterialized venous flow.[56] Unlike hemangiomas, AVMs do not have a well-defined soft tissue mass.[51] MRA can be used to depict the vascular anatomy, extent, and number of feeding arteries, thereby facilitating treatment planning. Time-resolved MRA can be used to depict the flow characteristics (high flow vs low flow) within the AVM as well as feeding arteries and the characteristic rapid venous drainage.[51]

Hypothenar Hammer Syndrome

The hypothenar hammer syndrome is caused by chronic posttraumatic vascular insufficiency due to repetitive blunt trauma (eg, from vibrating tools or motorcycle).[57] The superficial branch of the ulnar artery, which becomes the superficial palmar arch, is exposed to injury and external forces that compress the artery against the hook of the hamate bone.[51,57] Aneurysm formation, dissection, narrowing, and frank occlusion of the vessel can occur due to arterial intimal thickening. Intimal damage may lead to secondary thrombus formation with subsequent embolization of the second through fifths digits.[54]

MRA allows evaluating the integrity of the ulnar artery and its branches, defining the extent of vessel injury, and assessing the presence of collateral vessels.[1] It may demonstrate corkscrew elongation with alternating stenoses and ectasia of the ulnar artery.[51] In advanced cases, thrombosis and emboli are often seen.[58] Axial T1-weighted imaging might depict the thickened wall of the ulnar artery at the level of the hook of the hamate.[51] In some cases, the ulnar artery demonstrates complete segmental occlusion (**Fig. 10**). A history of repetitive trauma is essential to establish the diagnosis.

Raynaud Phenomenon

Raynaud phenomenon is characterized by peripheral arterial vasospasm of the digital arteries in response to cold or emotional stress. The vasospasm may dramatically reduce the blood flow, causing discoloration of the fingers, pain, and sensations of cold and/or numbness.[59] Raynaud phenomenon can be primary (idiopathic and referred to as Raynaud disease) or secondary to several different diseases, including rheumatologic diseases, such as scleroderma.[59]

MRA, through targeted imaging of the hand, can provide depiction of digital hyperemia, arterial stenosis, or complete vessel occlusion[1,60] and allows for treatment monitoring with vasodilators.[61]

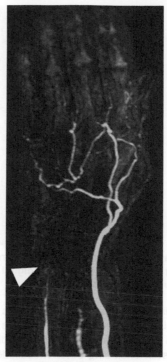

Fig. 10. Hypothenar Hammer syndrome. Coronal MIP of contrast-enhanced 3-D time-resolved MRA demonstrates occlusion (*arrowhead*) of the right ulnar artery proximal to the origin of the superficial palmar arch.

MRA findings tend to be descriptive rather than pathognomonic and are characterized by gradual narrowing and tapering of the proper digital vessels, often with capillary congestion in the fingertips (**Fig. 11**).[2] The main clinical utility of MRA and conventional MR imaging sequences lies in the exclusion of other possible causes, such as vasculitides (**Fig. 12**) or distal embolic disease (**Fig. 13**).[1] It may be helpful to repeat time-resolved MRA before and after warming of the hand (warming packs work well) in an attempt to reverse vasospasm to help establish or exclude this diagnosis.

Thromboangiitis Obliterans

Thromboangiitis obliterans (also known as Buerger disease) is a chronic nonatherosclerotic endarteritis manifesting as inflammation and thrombosis of distal extremity small and medium-sized arteries and veins resulting in relapsing episodes of distal extremity ischemia.[62] It is closely related to tobacco use and may also occur with smokeless nicotine-containing products.[62] Patients may initially present with hand claudication, which can progresses to ulceration and even gangrene.[63]

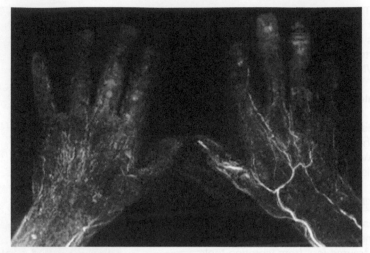

Fig. 11. Raynaud syndrome. MIP of non–contrast-enhanced flow-sensitive dephasing MRA demonstrates gradual narrowing and tapering of the distal digital vessels. The right hand is more affected and shows occlusions also at the level of the palmar arteries.

MRA may identify segmental stenoses or occlusions, collateral vessels adjacent to sites of occlusion, or a proximal source of embolic disease or may assist in excluding other vasculitides.[64,65] A corkscrew appearance of the digital arteries is often seen, although these findings are not pathognomonic for thromboangiitis obliterans. Therefore, MRA plays an important, albeit ancillary, role in establishing the diagnosis as well as

defining the extent and severity of disease. MRA is also helpful in excluding other vasculitides or identifying a proximal source of embolic disease.[1]

Benign and Malignant Tumors

Soft tissue tumors of the hand and wrist comprise approximately 15% and 4% of all benign and malignant soft tissue lesions, respectively.[66] A

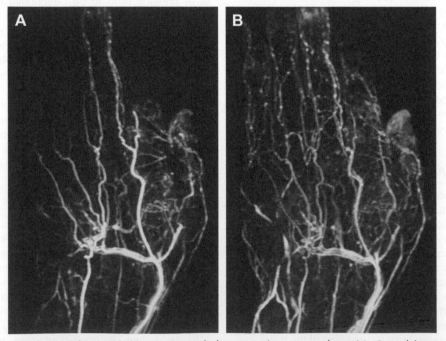

Fig. 12. Vasculitis in a patient with known Systemic lupus erythematosus, hepatitis C, and intravenous drug abuse. Coronal MIP of contrast-enhanced 3-D time-resolved MRA in the (*A*) early and (*B*) late arterial phases demonstrates delayed filling of the digital palmar arteries of the second, fourth, and fifths digit of the right hand and a beaded appearance of the distal arteries.

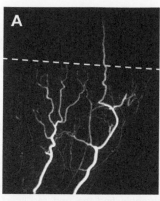
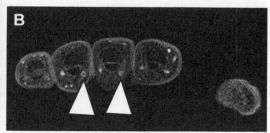

Fig. 13. Thromboembolic disease. (*A*) Coronal MIP of contrast-enhanced 3-D time-resolved arterial-phase MRA demonstrates filling defects within almost every digital palmar artery of the right hand except for the digital radial palmar artery of the second digit. (*B*) Axial delayed-phase fat-saturated T1-weighted imaging visualizes central filling defects (*arrowheads*) within the digital palmar arteries representing multiple thrombi. The dotted line (*A*) indicates the level of the section (*B*).

vast majority of soft tissue tumors of the upper extremity are benign.[67] Benign tumors include glomus tumors, tendon giant cell tumors, ganglion cysts, and Dupuytren contracture.[68] Malignant tumors are rare and include chondrosarcoma, osteosarcoma, synovial sarcoma, fibrosarcoma, and malignant vascular tumors.[69] Malignant tumors tend to be aggressive, invasive, and poorly circumscribed but may display a deceptively nonaggressive appearance on MR Imaging. Any lesion that does not satisfy the diagnostic criteria for the common benign lesions (outlined previously) warrants further work-up.

MRA may be used conjunction with conventional MR imaging sequences for characterizing the local extent and spread of the tumors as well as the relation of a tumor with normal vasculature. MRA can also be used to evaluate the vascular anatomy of tumors, including both arterial supply and venous drainage.[70] MR imaging cannot reliably distinguish malignant from benign tumors; in many circumstances, a specific diagnosis requires tissue sampling or taking into account the location of the lesion within the hand or wrist as well as its MR signal characteristics.[67]

SUMMARY

The MRA toolbox includes a wide array of versatile methods for diagnosis and therapy planning in patients with a variety of upper extremity vascular pathologies. MRA can provide excellent image quality with high spatial and high temporal resolution without the disadvantages of ionizing radiation, iodinated contrast, and operator dependency. The appropriate technique should be used and tailored for each individual to achieve optimal image quality and maximal diagnostic

yield. Contrast-enhanced techniques are generally preferred due to their robustness, image quality, and shorter scan times. Non–contrast-enhanced techniques may be helpful in patients with contraindications to gadolinium-based contrast agents but are generally less robust and more time consuming. Time-resolved CE-MRA is particularly helpful for the upper extremity because it provides both high spatial and high temporal resolution imaging and can be used to assess the hemodynamics of vascular disease. This article provides a basic overview of available MRA techniques and a description of the clinical entities that are well suited for evaluation with CE-MRA.

REFERENCES

1. Stepansky F, Hecht EM, Rivera R, et al. Dynamic MR angiography of upper extremity vascular disease: pictorial review. Radiographics 2008;28(1):e28.
2. Connell DA, Koulouris G, Thorn DA, et al. Contrast-enhanced MR angiography of the hand. Radiographics 2002;22(3):583–99.
3. Kramer JH, Grist TM. Peripheral MR Angiography. Magn Reson Imaging Clin N Am 2012;20(4):761–76.
4. Leiner T, Habets J, Versluis B, et al. Subtractionless first-pass single contrast medium dose peripheral MR angiography using two-point Dixon fat suppression. Eur Radiol 2013;23(8):2228–35.
5. Lee VS, Lee HM, Rofsky NM. Magnetic resonance angiography of the hand. A review. Invest Radiol 1998;33(9):687–98.
6. Thomson LK, Thomson PC, Kingsmore DB, et al. Diagnosing nephrogenic systemic fibrosis in the post-FDA restriction era. J Magn Reson Imaging 2015;41(5):1268–71.
7. Davenport MS, Cohan RH, Ellis JH. Contrast media controversies in 2015: imaging patients with renal

impairment or risk of contrast reaction. AJR Am J Roentgenol 2015;204(6):1174–81.

8. Bley TA, Duffek CC, Francois CJ, et al. Presurgical localization of the artery of Adamkiewicz with time-resolved 3.0-T MR angiography. Radiology 2010; 255(3):873–81.

9. Korosec FR, Frayne R, Grist TM, et al. Time-resolved contrast-enhanced 3D MR angiography. Magn Reson Med 1996;36(3):345–51.

10. Miyazaki M, Akahane M. Non-contrast enhanced MR angiography: established techniques. J Magn Reson Imaging 2012;35(1):1–19.

11. Wheaton AJ, Miyazaki M. Non-contrast enhanced MR angiography: physical principles. J Magn Reson Imaging 2012;36(2):286–304.

12. Morita S, Masukawa A, Suzuki K, et al. Unenhanced MR angiography: techniques and clinical applications in patients with chronic kidney disease. Radiographics 2011;31(2):E13–33.

13. Pelc NJ, Bernstein MA, Shimakawa A, et al. Encoding strategies for three-direction phase-contrast MR imaging of flow. J Magn Reson Imaging 1991;1(4): 405–13.

14. Klarhofer M, Csapo B, Balassy C, et al. High-resolution blood flow velocity measurements in the human finger. Magn Reson Med 2001;45(4):716–9.

15. Goyen M, Debatin JF. Gadopentetate dimeglumine-enhanced three-dimensional MR-angiography: dosing, safety, and efficacy. J Magn Reson Imaging 2004;19(3):261–73.

16. Veldhoen S, Behzadi C, Derlin T, et al. Exact monitoring of aortic diameters in Marfan patients without gadolinium contrast: intraindividual comparison of 2D SSFP imaging with 3D CE-MRA and echocardiography. Eur Radiol 2014;25(3):872–82.

17. Goyen M, Debatin JF. Gadobenate dimeglumine (MultiHance) for magnetic resonance angiography: review of the literature. Eur Radiol 2003;13(Suppl 3):N19–27.

18. Bannas P, Schiebler ML, Motosugi U, et al. Pulmonary MRA: differentiation of pulmonary embolism from truncation artefact. Eur Radiol 2014;24(8): 1942–9.

19. Scott LJ. Gadobutrol: a review of its use for contrast-enhanced magnetic resonance imaging in adults and children. Clin Drug Investig 2013; 33(4):303–14.

20. Sabach AS, Bruno M, Kim D, et al. Gadofosveset trisodium: abdominal and peripheral vascular applications. AJR Am J Roentgenol 2013;200(6):1378–86.

21. Prince MR. Body MR angiography with gadolinium contrast agents. Magn Reson Imaging Clin N Am 1996;4(1):11–24.

22. Reivich M, Holling HE, Roberts B, et al. Reversal of blood flow through the vertebral artery and its effect on cerebral circulation. N Engl J Med 1961; 265:878–85.

23. Potter BJ, Pinto DS. Subclavian steal syndrome. Circulation 2014;129(22):2320–3.

24. Shadman R, Criqui MH, Bundens WP, et al. Subclavian artery stenosis: prevalence, risk factors, and association with cardiovascular diseases. J Am Coll Cardiol 2004;44(3):618–23.

25. Huang BY, Castillo M. Radiological reasoning: extracranial causes of unilateral decreased brain perfusion. AJR Am J Roentgenol 2007;189(6 Suppl):S49–54.

26. de Souza AW, de Carvalho JF. Diagnostic and classification criteria of Takayasu arteritis. J Autoimmun 2014;48–49:79–83.

27. Park JH, Han MC, Kim SH, et al. Takayasu arteritis: angiographic findings and results of angioplasty. AJR Am J Roentgenol 1989;153(5):1069–74.

28. Alibaz-Oner F, Aydin SZ, Direskeneli H. Advances in the diagnosis, assessment and outcome of Takayasu's arteritis. Clin Rheumatol 2013;32(5):541–6.

29. Ness T, Bley TA, Schmidt WA, et al. The diagnosis and treatment of giant cell arteritis. Dtsch Arztebl Int 2013;110(21):376–85 [quiz: 386].

30. Espigol-Frigole G, Prieto-Gonzalez S, Alba MA, et al. Advances in the diagnosis of large vessel vasculitis. Rheum Dis Clin North Am 2015;41(1):125–40.

31. Klink T, Geiger J, Both M, et al. Giant cell arteritis: diagnostic accuracy of MR imaging of superficial cranial arteries in initial diagnosis-results from a multicenter trial. Radiology 2014;273(3):844–52.

32. Markl M, Uhl M, Wieben O, et al. High resolution 3T MRI for the assessment of cervical and superficial cranial arteries in giant cell arteritis. J Magn Reson Imaging 2006;24(2):423–7.

33. Geiger J, Bley T, Uhl M, et al. Diagnostic value of T2-weighted imaging for the detection of superficial cranial artery inflammation in giant cell arteritis. J Magn Reson Imaging 2010;31(2):470–4.

34. Ferrante MA. The thoracic outlet syndromes. Muscle Nerve 2012;45(6):780–95.

35. Ersoy H, Steigner ML, Coyner KB, et al. Vascular thoracic outlet syndrome: protocol design and diagnostic value of contrast-enhanced 3D MR angiography and equilibrium phase imaging on 1.5- and 3-T MRI scanners. AJR Am J Roentgenol 2012; 198(5):1180–7.

36. Aralasmak A, Cevikol C, Karaali K, et al. MRI findings in thoracic outlet syndrome. Skeletal Radiol 2012;41(11):1365–74.

37. Engelberger RP, Kucher N. Management of deep vein thrombosis of the upper extremity. Circulation 2012;126(6):768–73.

38. Grant JD, Stevens SM, Woller SC, et al. Diagnosis and management of upper extremity deep-vein thrombosis in adults. Thromb Haemost 2012;108(6):1097–108.

39. Sampson FC, Goodacre SW, Thomas SM, et al. The accuracy of MRI in diagnosis of suspected deep vein thrombosis: systematic review and meta-analysis. Eur Radiol 2007;17(1):175–81.

40. Schiebler ML, Nagle SK, Francois CJ, et al. Effectiveness of MR angiography for the primary diagnosis of acute pulmonary embolism: clinical outcomes at 3 months and 1 year. J Magn Reson Imaging 2013;38(4):914–25.

41. Ruehm SG, Zimny K, Debatin JF. Direct contrast-enhanced 3D MR venography. Eur Radiol 2001; 11(1):102–12.

42. Rohrer M, Bauer H, Mintorovitch J, et al. Comparison of magnetic properties of MRI contrast media solutions at different magnetic field strengths. Invest Radiol 2005;40(11):715–24.

43. Achneck HE, Sileshi B, Li M, et al. Surgical aspects and biological considerations of arteriovenous fistula placement. Semin Dial 2010;23(1):25–33.

44. Rose DA, Sonaike E, Hughes K. Hemodialysis access. Surg Clin North Am 2013;93(4):997–1012, x.

45. Planken RN, Tordoir JH, Dammers R, et al. Stenosis detection in forearm hemodialysis arteriovenous fistulae by multiphase contrast-enhanced magnetic resonance angiography: preliminary experience. J Magn Reson Imaging 2003;17(1):54–64.

46. Zhang J, Hecht EM, Maldonado T, et al. Time-resolved 3D MR angiography with parallel imaging for evaluation of hemodialysis fistulas and grafts: initial experience. AJR Am J Roentgenol 2006; 186(5):1436–42.

47. Smits JH, Bos C, Elgersma OE, et al. Hemodialysis access imaging: comparison of flow-interrupted contrast-enhanced MR angiography and digital subtraction angiography. Radiology 2002;225(3):829–34.

48. Broome DR, Cottrell AC, Kanal E. Response to "Will dialysis prevent the development of nephrogenic systemic fibrosis after gadolinium-based contrast administration?". AJR Am J Roentgenol 2007; 189(4):W234–5.

49. Joffe P, Thomsen HS, Meusel M. Pharmacokinetics of gadodiamide injection in patients with severe renal insufficiency and patients undergoing hemodialysis or continuous ambulatory peritoneal dialysis. Acad Radiol 1998;5(7):491–502.

50. ACR Manual on Contrast Media. 2013.

51. Drape JL, Feydy A, Guerini H, et al. Vascular lesions of the hand. Eur J Radiol 2005;56(3):331–43.

52. Wassef M, Enjolras O. Superficial vascular malformations: classification and histopathology. Ann Pathol 1999;19(3):253–64 [in French].

53. Ek ET, Suh N, Carlson MG. Vascular anomalies of the hand and wrist. J Am Acad Orthop Surg 2014;22(6): 352–60.

54. Yakes WF. Angiographic and interventional procedures in the hand. Philadelphia: WB Saunders Company; 1996.

55. Kransdorf MM, MD. Imaging of soft tissue tumors. Philadelphia: Lippicott Williams & Wilkins; 2013.

56. Rak KM, Yakes WF, Ray RL, et al. MR imaging of symptomatic peripheral vascular malformations. AJR Am J Roentgenol 1992;159(1):107–12.

57. Duncan WC. Hypothenar hammer syndrome: an uncommon cause of digital ischemia. J Am Acad Dermatol 1996;34(5 Pt 2):880–3.

58. Winterer JT, Ghanem N, Roth M, et al. Diagnosis of the hypothenar hammer syndrome by high-resolution contrast-enhanced MR angiography. Eur Radiol 2002;12(10):2457–62.

59. Maverakis E, Patel F, Kronenberg DG, et al. International consensus criteria for the diagnosis of Raynaud's phenomenon. J Autoimmun 2014; 48–49:60–5.

60. Walcher J, Strecker R, Goldacker S, et al. High resolution 3 Tesla contrast-enhanced MR angiography of the hands in Raynaud's disease. Clin Rheumatol 2007;26(4):587–9.

61. Park JK, Park EA, Lee W, et al. Baseline MRA predicts the treatment response to vasodilator udenafil in patients with secondary Raynaud's phenomenon. Clin Exp Rheumatol 2014;32(6 Suppl 86):167–70.

62. Wu W, Chaer RA. Nonarteriosclerotic vascular disease. Surg Clin North Am 2013;93(4):833–75, viii.

63. Piazza G, Creager MA. Thromboangiitis obliterans. Circulation 2010;121(16):1858–61.

64. Shah DJ, Brown B, Kim RJ, et al. Magnetic resonance evaluation of peripheral arterial disease. Magn Reson Imaging Clin N Am 2007;15(4): 653–79, vii.

65. Dimmick SJ, Goh AC, Cauzza E, et al. Imaging appearances of Buerger's disease complications in the upper and lower limbs. Clin Radiol 2012; 67(12):1207–11.

66. Kransdorf MJ, Murphey MD. MR imaging of musculoskeletal tumors of the hand and wrist. Magn Reson Imaging Clin N Am 1995;3(2):327–44.

67. Teh J, Whiteley G. MRI of soft tissue masses of the hand and wrist. Br J Radiol 2007;80(949): 47–63.

68. Dewan AK, Chhabra AB, Khanna AJ, et al. Magnetic resonance imaging of the hand and wrist: techniques and spectrum of disease: AAOS exhibit selection. J Bone Joint Surg Am 2013;95(10):e68.

69. Wong JC, Abraham JA. Upper extremity considerations for oncologic surgery. Orthop Clin North Am 2014;45(4):541–64.

70. Peterson JJ, Bancroft LW, Kransdorf MJ. Principles of tumor imaging. Eur J Radiol 2005;56(3):319–30.

Key MR Imaging Features of Common Hand Surgery Conditions

Tristan de Mooij, MD[a,b], Scott Riester, MD[b],
Sanjeev Kakar, MD, MRCS[b],*

KEYWORDS

- MR imaging • Scaphoid fractures • Hand infections • Scapholunate ligament
- Triangular fibrocartilage complex • Ulnar collateral ligament of the thumb

KEY POINTS

- Deep-space infections may occur in the potential spaces of the hand. Allied to clinical examination, MR imaging can visualize fluid collections and the spread of tissue inflammation.
- MR imaging can diagnose occult scaphoid fractures, whereas other imaging studies often present false negative in the acute stage. It can also aid in the detection of scaphoid proximal pole viability after a fracture.
- MR imaging is useful in diagnosing scapholunate ligament tears when features are not yet apparent on radiographs; MR imaging can assess cartilage damage and, thus, direct treatment.
- MR imaging of the thumb can help detect an ulnar collateral ligament injury and also the presence of a concomitant Stener lesion.
- MR imaging can help with the diagnosis of complete, transverse ulnotriquetral ligament tears and foveal disruption of the triangular fibrocartilage complex with high sensitivity and specificity; however, longitudinal tears may present with more subtle imaging features and subsequently sensitivity ranges between 30% and 58%, with 60% specificity.

INTRODUCTION

Common hand injuries like scaphoid fractures, scapholunate (SL) ligament injuries, and triangular fibrocartilage complex (TFCC) tears are typically caused by a fall onto the outstretched hand. In the acute setting, patients may present with vague signs and symptoms, and specific tests during physical examination have a limited specificity to distinguish the myriad of pathologic conditions. Although the radiological workup starts with plain radiographs, these can lack the sensitivity to detect certain soft tissue injuries, such as a SL ligament or TFCC damage. The advent of improved MR imaging technology and dedicated wrist coils has allowed for unique opportunities to visualize subtle soft tissue damage as well as concomitant injuries.

This article discusses common hand conditions, including deep-space infections, scaphoid fracture, SL ligament tears, ulnar collateral ligament (UCL) injuries of the thumb metacarpophalangeal (MCP) joint, and ulnotriquetral ligament (UTL) tears, and focuses on the imaging findings and the utility of MR imaging in their diagnosis and management.

The authors have nothing of value to disclose that is relevant to this article.
[a] Department of Neurologic Surgery, Mayo Clinic, 200 First Street Southwest, Rochester, MN 55905, USA;
[b] Department of Orthopedic Surgery, Mayo Clinic, 200 First Street Southwest, Rochester, MN 55905, USA
* Corresponding author.
E-mail address: Kakar.Sanjeev@mayo.edu

mri.theclinics.com

DEEP-SPACE INFECTION OF THE HAND
Anatomy

The deep spaces in the hand and forearm include the thenar, midpalmar, hypothenar, and Parona space (**Fig. 1**).

Infections in closed cavities or tunnels result in the accumulation of exudates or pus and the establishment of high pressures within the compartments. This state can lead to a reduction of blood flow, regional anoxia, hypoperfusion, and a deficient immune response. The increase in compartmental pressure leads to the expansion of the ischemic zone and facilitates the dissemination of the infection.[1–4] Thenar space infections are the most common deep-space infections and, if not promptly treated, can spread to the dorsal side of the hand after invading the fascia of the adductor pollicis muscles. A Parona space infection may be isolated or may result from contiguous spread from ruptured radial or ulnar bursae. Such a rupture can involve the midpalmar space and form a horseshoe abscess.[5] Infections to the thenar and midpalmar space may be caused by adjacent infections, such as a superficial abscess or a flexor tenosynovitis.[6]

Imaging

Deep-space infections are diagnosed by physical examination, with the examiner attempting to elicit induration, fluctuance, and the clinical signs of suppurative flexor tenosynovitis: fusiform swelling, pain with passive extension, pain with palpation along the tendon sheath, and a finger held in slight flexion.[4] The distinction between cellulitis, abscess, and flexor tenosynovitis can still be difficult by physical examination alone, but radiographs, ultrasound, and MR imaging can provide critical additional information. Radiographs should be taken in all cases presenting with hand infections to rule out foreign bodies, gas, and chronic osteomyelitis.

Differential Diagnosis

Suspected deep-space infections need to be discerned from flexor tenosynovitis, superficial abscess, and osteomyelitis (**Fig. 2**). Abscess cavities are most often spherical or elliptical and may contain debris, septae, or gas with the liquefied contents demonstrating a range of echogenicity. Abscess formation can complicate cellulitis and is seen with MR imaging as an intermediate- to

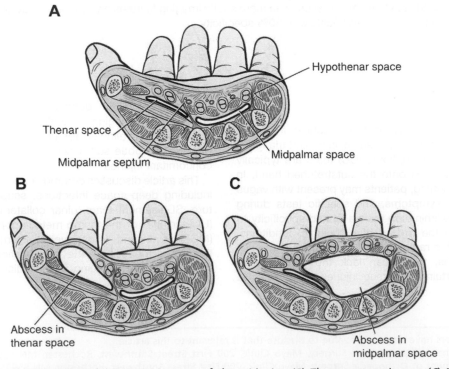

Fig. 1. Deep palmar spaces. (*A*) Potential spaces of the midpalm. (*B*) Thenar space abscess. (*C*) Midpalmar space abscess. (*From* Stevanovic MV, Sharpe S. Acute infections. In: Green DP, Hotchkiss RN, Pederson WC, et al, editors. Green's operative hand surgery. 5th edition. Philadelphia: Churchill Livingstone; 2005. p. 71; with permission.)

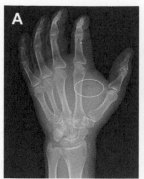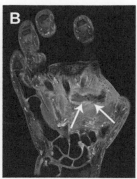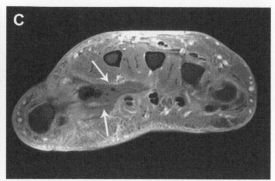

Fig. 2. (A) Radiography of the hand shows air bubbles (oval) within the soft tissue of the first interspace. (B) Coronal T1-weighted spoiled gradient recalled (SPGR) image with fat suppression after intravenous contrast shows a nonenhancing fluid collection (arrows) containing low-signal air bubbles, consistent with an abscess with gas. (C) Axial T1-weighted SPGR image with fat suppression shows the abscess (arrows) with central air bubbles. The MR image shows that the adjacent tendons and bone are not affected.

low-signal-intensity focal lesion on T1-weighted images, with uniform to slightly heterogeneous high signal intensity on fluid-sensitive images and a peripheral rim of enhancement on postcontrast images. Given the intimate relationship of the midpalmar and the thenar spaces, any infection persisting for a prolonged period of time can extend into the adjacent space.

Treatment

Drainage and thorough irrigation of deep-space infections is typically the first step in surgical management. Nonviable tissue should be sharply debrided. Patients are placed on antibiotics and may need additional surgical procedures to eradicate the infection.

SCAPHOID FRACTURE
Anatomy

The scaphoid has a complex 3-dimensional geometry that encompasses a proximal pole, waist, and distal pole. It serves as an important link between the proximal and the distal carpal row and is almost entirely covered in articular cartilage. Although the dorsal branch of the superficial radial artery provides dual vascularity to the distal pole and the tubercle, the proximal pole is vascularized via retrograde endosteal branches.[7] Because of the paucity of the vascularity, fracture displacement, and the restriction to primary bone healing caused by the absence of periosteum, the scaphoid has a high risk of nonunion and avascular necrosis.[8]

Pathogenesis

The typical mechanism of injury involves a fall onto an outstretched wrist in an extended and radial deviated manner. Although 70% to 80% of all fractures occur at the waist, 10% to 20% occur at the proximal pole and 5% involve the tubercle and distal pole. After a fracture, the proximal pole tends to extend given its attachment to the lunate by the SL ligament and the distal fragment flexes because of the scaphotrapezial forces resulting in a possible humpback deformity. Scaphoid fractures are commonly classified according to the Herbert classification[9] (Fig. 3).

Imaging

Initial imaging studies for a suspected scaphoid fracture include posteroanterior radiographs with the wrist in ulnar deviation, semipronated, and semisupinated 45 oblique views, and a lateral view. The posteroanterior view in ulnar deviation extends the scaphoid, thereby allowing it to be imaged along its longitudinal axis. The semipronated view visualizes the waist and distal-third region, whereas the semisupinated view visualizes the dorsal ridge. The lateral view may demonstrate a waist fracture, fracture displacement, and angulation. Treatment is guided by fracture stability and displacement, which are determined by the following criteria: (1) 1-mm displacement, (2) greater than 10 angular displacement, (3) fracture comminution, (4) greater than 15 of radiolunate angulation, (5) greater than 60 SL angulation, and (6) greater than 35 intrascaphoid angulation. As radiographs tend to underestimate true displacement, a visible fracture line on plain radiographs should be considered a displaced fracture.[10]

When the clinical presentation and examination are suspicious for a scaphoid fracture but the radiographs are inconclusive, advanced imaging is warranted[11–13] (Fig. 4). MR imaging is used to

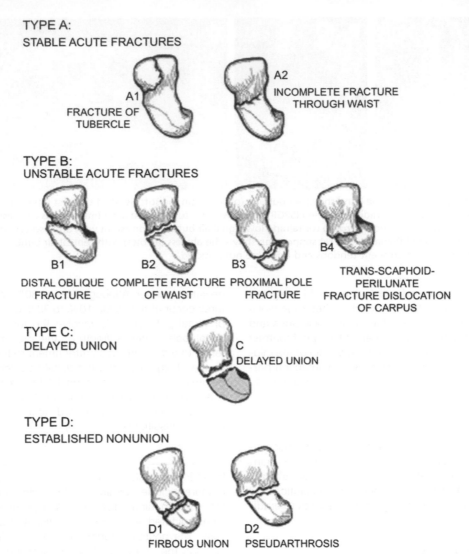

TYPE A:
STABLE ACUTE FRACTURES

A1
FRACTURE OF
TUBERCLE

A2
INCOMPLETE FRACTURE
THROUGH WAIST

TYPE B:
UNSTABLE ACUTE FRACTURES

B1
DISTAL OBLIQUE
FRACTURE

B2
COMPLETE FRACTURE
OF WAIST

B3
PROXIMAL POLE
FRACTURE

B4
TRANS-SCAPHOID-
PERILUNATE
FRACTURE DISLOCATION
OF CARPUS

TYPE C:
DELAYED UNION

C
DELAYED UNION

TYPE D:
ESTABLISHED NONUNION

D1
FIRBOUS UNION

D2
PSEUDARTHROSIS

Fig. 3. The Herbert classification. (*From* Herbert TJ. The fractured scaphoid. St Louis (MO): Quality Medical Publishing; 1990. p. 52; with permission.)

detect these occult injuries given its high sensitivity and specificity as well as its ability to detect additional injuries. With the addition of gadolinium enhancement, the MR imaging can help to assess for proximal pole viability.[14–17] Obtaining early MR imaging has been shown to be more cost-effective than 2 weeks of expectative splinting and repeated evaluation, improves the opportunity for a timely intervention, and reduces visits.[16,18]

Assessment of the viability of the proximal pole plays a central role in predicting treatment outcomes. Although MR imaging cannot measure the actual blood flow, it may evaluate edema as a derivative of proximal pole viability[19,20] (**Fig. 5**). Therefore, MR imaging has become useful to assess viability despite accuracy rates of 68% of conventional MR imaging

and 83% of gadolinium-enhanced MR imaging.[19,20] Care needs to be exerted when interpreting the MR imaging; preserved marrow in the proximal pole of the scaphoid or mummified fat may yield a high T1 signal that could be mistaken for a measure of scaphoid viability.[11] In addition, contrast-enhanced MR imaging may give false-positive results for fragment viability, for example, by invagination of fibrous tissue impeding the impregnation of the proximal pole.[21,22] False-positive results may be the result of contrast diffusion into the necrotic fracture fragment caused by a 4- to 9-minute delay between contrast administration and imaging.[21,23] The gold standard to determine proximal pole viability continues to be intraoperative presence of punctate bleeding.

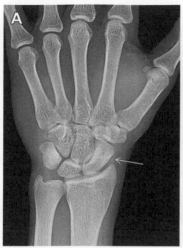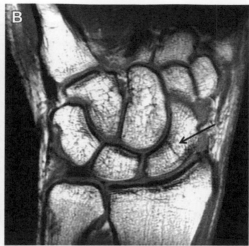

Fig. 4. (*A*) Radiograph of the hand obtained immediately after a fall on an outstretched hand is negative for fracture. There is subtle soft tissue density replacing the normal scaphoid fat stripe (*white arrow*). (*B*) Coronal T1-weighted MR image obtained 1 day later shows a low-signal, horizontal nondisplaced scaphoid fracture (*black arrow*).

Differential Diagnosis

Suspected scaphoid fractures need to be discerned from a possible SL injury, wrist sprain, wrist contusion, fracture of other carpal bones, and distal radius fracture.

Treatment

Nonoperative treatment is indicated for nondisplaced acute fractures of the distal pole, with healing typically seen by 6 to 8 weeks.[24,25] Evidence concerning optimal treatment of acute nondisplaced or minimally displaced waist fracture is less clear. Studies have reported a 98% union with conservative treatment of nondisplaced fractures over the course of 8 to 12 weeks.[26] However, cast treatment has a longer immobilization time, joint stiffness, reduced grip strength, and longer time to return to manual work. In comparison, operative treatment is associated with a 5-week reduction in union time and a 7-week reduction in return to work[27] (**Fig. 6**). Fractures of the proximal pole are best treated surgically as these are at high risk of going onto a nonunion. Surgical treatment is also indicated for unstable or displaced fractures and those that present on a delayed basis because of their higher risk of nonunion.

Scaphoid fractures require, at minimum, serial radiographs in order to assess fracture line obliteration and trabeculation of the fracture site.[28] MR imaging will continue to show an abnormal signal around a stable fracture even as healing progresses to union. A double line representing the fracture line coupled with the revascularization front signifies healing on MR imaging; failure of this front to advance is almost always associated with eventual nonunion.[29] Fracture union on MR imaging is only definitively shown by the presence of normal signal intensity marrow crossing the previous fracture line on T1-weighed images.[30,31] Postoperative MR imaging may become a technically demanding procedure because of the artifacts from the use of metal instruments and Kirschner wires, even after their removal.[32,33] Therefore, historically, the MR imaging scan is most often used to identify the presence of a scaphoid fracture and vascularity of the proximal pole to rule out avascular necrosis rather than to determine its healing.

SCAPHOLUNATE INTEROSSEOUS LIGAMENT TEAR

Anatomy

To keep the proximal carpal row in neutral rotation, the SL, lunotriquetral ligaments, and the extrinsic carpal ligaments provide stability. The SL is a C-shaped structure consisting of a stronger dorsal ligamentous portion (2–3 mm thick), a volar ligamentous portion (1 mm thick), and a proximal fibrocartilaginous membranous portion.[34]

Pathogenesis

SL instability, a form of carpal instability dissociative, is a common cause of carpal instability. Its disruption occurs when the wrist is loaded in extension, supination, and ulnar deviation.[35] Torn

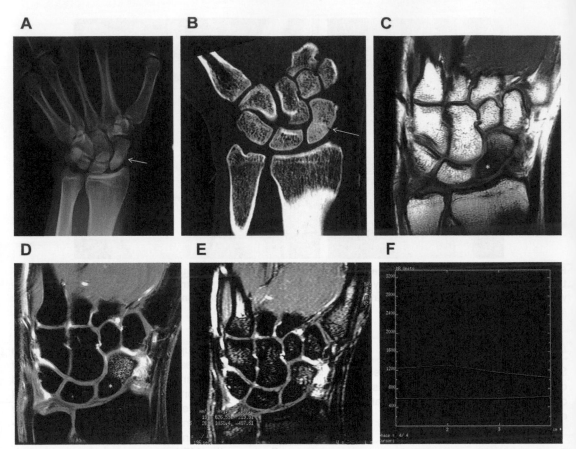

Fig. 5. (*A*) Radiograph of a chronically ununited scaphoid waist fractures (*arrow*) shows increased density in the proximal pole fragment, worrisome for avascular necrosis (AVN). (*B*) Coronal reformatted computed tomography image shows sclerosis in the proximal pole with some preservation of trabecular architecture. The fracture is again seen (*arrow*). (*C*) Coronal T1-weighted MR image without contrast demonstrates the replacement of normal marrow fat in the proximal pole of the scaphoid (*asterisk*) with less complete replacement of the distal pole. (*D*) Delayed postcontrast T1-weighted spoiled gradient recalled coronal image with fat suppression shows no enhancement in the proximal pole (*asterisk*) but some enhancement by diffusion in the distal pole of the scaphoid. (*E*) Compound dynamic image with analysis. The encircled area shows avascularity of the proximal scaphoid. (*F*) shows no enhancement of the proximal pole on any phase, consistent with AVN. The normal capitate was evaluated for comparison.

ligaments allow for pathologic displacement and rotatory instabilities that can cause degenerative arthritis within the wrist. SL injuries typically occur at the bone-ligament interface of the scaphoid and can range from partial to complete tears. Isolated injuries to the SL, in which the secondary stabilizers of the carpus remain intact, can result in predynamic or dynamic instability where the scaphoid is normally aligned with the lunate. When the secondary stabilizers, such as the dorsal intercarpal and scapho-trapezoid-trapezium ligaments, become attenuated, the scaphoid tends to flex and the lunate extends to give dorsal intercarpal segment instability.[36] The altered carpal kinematics that may ensue can result in the development of degenerative changes in the radiocarpal and midcarpal joints, the so-called SL advanced

collapse. As the scaphoid pronates within the scaphoid fossa, degeneration is seen first within the radioscaphoid joint and gradually progresses within the capitolunate joint leading to midcarpal arthritis. The radiolunate joint is typically spared.

Imaging

Although arthroscopy is considered the gold standard to diagnose SL ligament tears, the functional gold standard is a combination of history, physical examination, radiographs, and MR imaging. Bilateral anteroposterior and lateral radiographs, combined with pronated grip anteroposterior views, may reveal the following findings suggestive of complete SL tears: (1) Terry Thomas sign: a diastasis of the SL interval of 3 mm or greater

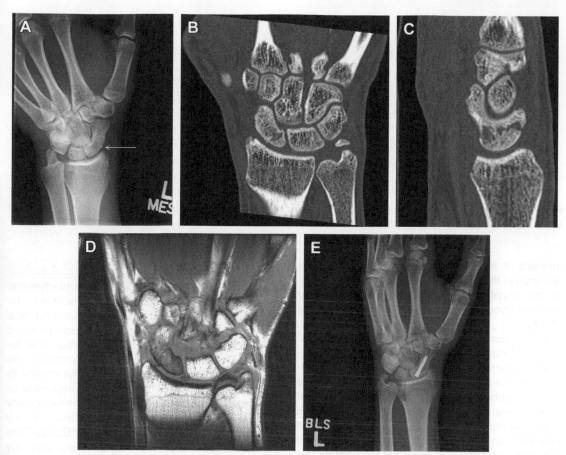

Fig. 6. A proximal pole fracture with subtle displacement on (*A*) scaphoid view on radiography, (*B,C*) Computed tomography, (*D*) Magnetic resonance imaging. Plain radiography showing fracture fixation at follow up (*E*).

or double the width of the SL interval in combination with a normal capitolunate interval[37]; (2) angular changes: SL angle of 60 or greater (normal 30–60), capitolunate angle of 15 or greater (normal 15 to 15), and radiolunate angle of 10 or greater (normal 10 to 10); (3) signet ring sign: excessive scaphoid flexion secondary to SL ligament instability[37,38]; (4) quadrangular lunate: extension of the lunate causes a rectangular appearance on posteroanterior radiographs; (5) disruption of Gilula lines: disruption of the smooth curvature between the proximal and midcarpal rows. However, in the acute setting, radiographs may give a false-negative appearance. Since the introduction of 3-T MR imaging scanners and dedicated wrist coils, 86% sensitivity and 100% specificity has been reported with MR imaging.[39] Additionally, MR imaging can provide valuable information on the degree of cartilage degeneration.

Differential Diagnosis

Suspected SL interosseous ligament (SLIL) injuries need to be discerned from scaphoid fracture or nonunion, scaphotrapezial arthritis, radiocarpal arthritis, de Quervain tenosynovitis, dorsal ganglion cyst, dorsal wrist impaction syndrome, perilunate instability, and isolated dorsal intercarpal ligament tears.[40]

Partial tears typically involve disruption of some of the SL ligament complex, such as the membranous or palmar structures[41] (**Figs. 7–9**). Injury to the SL ligament usually begins in the palmar component of the ligament, which is less stout than the dorsal component. The injury then progresses dorsally until a complete tear is present.[42] Secondary findings, such as the presence of excessive midcarpal joint fluid and associated ganglia/synovitis, may indicate a tear.[41]

Complete tears are diagnosed when there is a distinct area of discontinuity with increased signal

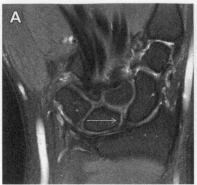
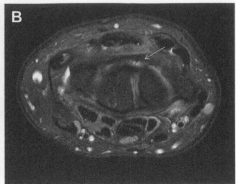

Fig. 7. Coronal (*A*) and axial (*B*) T2-weighted MR images with fat suppression show a tear of the dorsal portion of the SL ligament with an associated ganglion cyst (*arrow*).

intensity on fluid-sensitive sequences or complete absence of the ligament.[43] Severe distortion of ligament morphology, such as fraying, thinning, or abnormal course, may additionally be suggestive of a tear.[44]

A common source of misinterpretation of a tear is the contrast between the low-signal fibrocartilaginous attachment of the SL ligament in comparison with the high-signal articular hyaline cartilage of the scaphoid. Even so, false-positive bilateral findings are found in 75% to 90% of patients with unilateral complaints.[45–47] As complete intrinsic ligament tears often do not have evidence of carpal instability, it is important to correlate this potential finding with the extrinsic ligaments.[48]

Magnetic resonance (MR) arthrography (MRA) is useful to demonstrate pathologic communication between the midcarpal and radiocarpal joints within the wrist (**Fig. 10**). Lee and colleagues[49] found 91.7% to 95.8% accuracy of MRA in detecting SL ligament tears. MRA has the potential to increasingly detect these injuries given its relative low cost and minimal invasiveness.

Treatment

SL ligament injuries associated with predynamic instability may respond to cast treatment for 6 weeks. There are a myriad of different surgical options ranging from arthroscopic reduction and percutaneous pinning to limited partial wrist fusions. Key questions to ask in determining the type of surgical treatment include the chronicity of the injury, whether the ligament is reparable or not, the alignment of the scaphoid, the reducibility of the SL interval, and the development of any posttraumatic arthritis. The article by Garcia-Elias and colleagues[50] provides an excellent overview to the spectrum of available surgical treatments.

ULNAR COLLATERAL LIGAMENT OF THE THUMB TEAR
Anatomy

The true and accessory collateral ligaments provide ligamentous support to the MCP joint of the thumb. The true accessory ligaments arise from

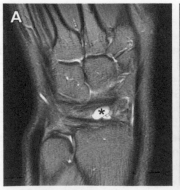
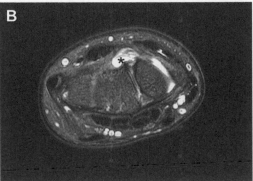

Fig. 8. Coronal (*A*) and axial (*B*) T2-weighted MR images with fat suppression show a more extensive tear of the dorsal and membranous portions of the SLIL with a large associated ganglion cyst (*asterisk*).

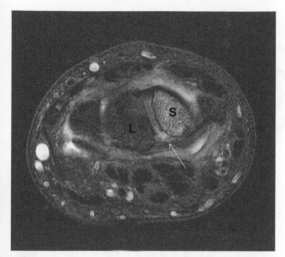

Fig. 9. Axial T2-weighted MR image with fat suppression shows a partial tear of the volar portion of the SLIL (*arrow*) after fall on an outstretched hand. Note edema in the scaphoid (S). The lunate (L) is normal.

the condyles of the metacarpal and pass obliquely to insert on the volar third of the proximal phalanx. The accessory collateral ligaments originate slightly more volar from the true collateral ligament and insert on the volar plate and the sesamoid bones. Secondary stabilizers to coronal plane deformity include the adductor pollicis, which inserts on the ulnar sesamoid, and the flexor pollicis brevis, which inserts on the radial sesamoid. Both muscles have secondary insertions onto the extensor mechanism via the adductor and abductor aponeuroses in order to provide additional lateral stability. Sagittal plane stability is provided by the stout dorsal capsule and fibrocartilage volar plate.

Pathogenesis

The UCL of the thumb MCP is usually torn by forceful abduction and extension of the thumb, thereby applying a radial force on the thumb MCP joint that can occur during a fall, athletic injury, or high-speed trauma. The UCL typically avulses from its insertion, but tears in its midsubstance or avulsions off of the metacarpal may occur.[51] Avulsions may coincide with midsubstance tears or involve the articular surface. Volar subluxation may ensue because of a supination rotation around the intact radial collateral ligament.[52] Ligament tears off the proximal phalanx may be complicated by interposition of the adductor aponeurosis, termed a *Stener lesion*, preventing healing of the ligament to its insertion[51] (**Fig. 11**). Other potentially associated injuries include tears of the dorsal capsule, volar plate, and the adductor aponeurosis. Chronic instability of the UCL, termed *gamekeeper's thumb*,[53] may be caused by inadequate treatment of an acute tear, failure to recognize a Stener lesion, or chronic repetitive attenuation.[53]

Imaging

Despite their recognized limitations, clinical examination and plain/stress radiographs remain the

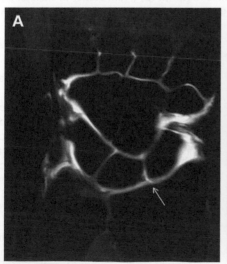
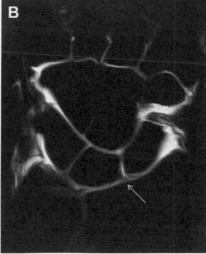

Fig. 10. (*A*) Coronal T1-weighted MR image with fat suppression in the presence of intra-articular gadolinium (MRA) shows contrast (*arrow*) extending from the radiocarpal joint to the SL interval, consistent with a complete tear. The contrast was introduced via a radiocarpal injection. (*B*) Coronal T2-weighted MR image with fat suppression in the presence of intra-articular contrast shows the high signal in the interval (*arrow*), but the communication with the joint is not as well seen as on the T1-weighted image, where gadolinium is bright.

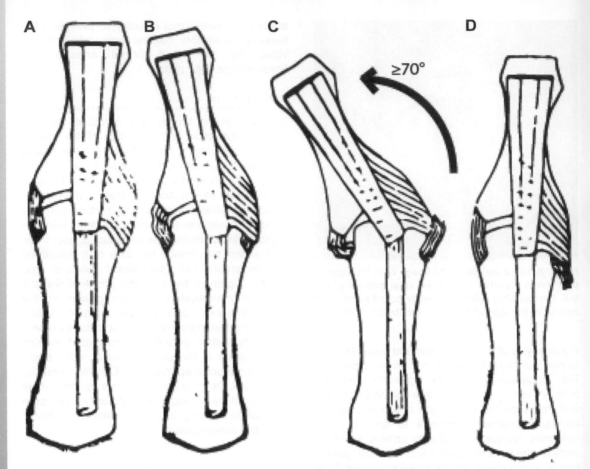

Fig. 11. The pathophysiology of the Stener lesion. From left to right, an axially neutral thumb MCP joint is stressed radially causing a complete UCL tear (*A-C*). When the thumb returns to its neutral position, the adductor aponeurosis is interposed between the avulsion fragment and its insertion on the proximal phalanx. This "stener" lesion thereby prevents healing of the UCL to its anatomic footprint (*D*) (*From* Stener B. Skeletal injuries associated with rupture of the ulnar collateral ligament of the metacarpophalangeal joint of the thumb. A clinical and anatomical study. Acta Chir Scand 1963;125:583–6.)

baseline tools used to evaluate acute UCL injury and guide management. Laxity greater than 35 in 30 flexion *or* greater than 15 difference in valgus in comparison with the uninjured thumb is suggestive of a true UCL injury with possible dorsal capsule disruption. Laxity greater than 35 in MCP joint extension is suggestive of an accessory UCL and volar plate injury.[54,55] Volar subluxation of the MCP joint is additionally suggestive of a complete tear with dorsal capsule disruption. The presence of fullness or a palpable mass on the ulnar aspect of the metacarpal head and neck is suggestive of a Stener lesion[54] (**Fig. 12**). Standard posteroanterior, lateral, and oblique radiographs should be obtained in all patients with suspected UCL injury to identify accompanying avulsions or condylar fractures. Stress radiographs may aid in the detection of instability but are associated

with a 25% false-negative rate and may displace the fracture.[56]

Although ultrasound has considerable value in evaluating UCL injury, its sensitivity and specificity are inferior to MR imaging as the technique remains highly operator dependent. Hergan and Mittler[57] examined the diagnostic accuracy of ultrasound with intraoperative findings in 39 patients with suspected UCL tears. In 36 cases, the ultrasound imaging correctly predicted the surgical findings, which included 16 Stener lesions.[57] Susic and colleagues[58] correctly identified only 2 of 5 Stener lesions in their cohort and reported an incorrect diagnosis of location of the ligament in 7 of 14 patients. Taken together, these studies obtained 76% sensitivity, 81% specificity, 81% accuracy, and 74% positive predictive value of ultrasound to detect these injuries. Hergan and

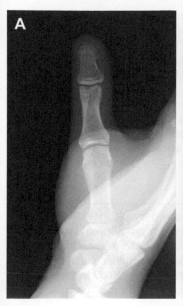

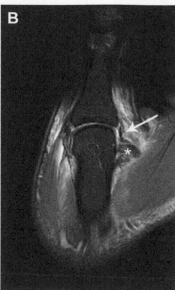

Fig. 12. (*A*) Roberts view of the thumb after a skiing injury is normal. (*B*) Coronal T2-weighted MR image with fat suppression of the thumb shows the completely torn and retracted ulnar collateral ligament (*asterisk*), which extends superficial to the aponeurosis (*arrow*), consistent with a Stener lesion. There is no bony avulsion in this case, which accounts for the normal radiograph.

colleagues[59] compared ultrasound and MR imaging and imaged 17 patients before surgical exploration. Two of 17 patients had misinterpretation of displacement of the UCL on ultrasound, whereas MR imaging was 100% specific and sensitive. Harper and colleagues[56] evaluated 19 patients, 5 of which received MR imaging and 14 MRAs. MRA resulted in 1 false-positive interpretation out of 14.

Romano and colleagues[60] used high-resolution MR imaging to characterize the detailed appearance of the thumb UCL after injury and suggested 5 distinct subclasses of ligament tear, including a partial tear, a Stener lesion, and avulsions fractures that were nondisplaced, minimally displaced (3 mm), and moderately displaced (3 mm). Milner and colleagues[61] have proposed a modification of the Romano classification system, defining their groups as partial tears/sprains, undisplaced (<3 mm), displaced (>3 mm), and Stener lesion (**Table 1**). This system, in their cohort, accurately identified the need for surgery (group 3 and 4) and those benefiting from conservative treatment (group 1 and 2).[61] Patients presenting with greater than 20% of the articular surface were treated as a fracture rather than a UCL injury and were, thus, excluded. Out of the 43 patients, 14 (33%) had a type 1 injury, 5 had a type 2 injury (12%), 10 had a type 3 injury (24%), and 14 had a type 4 injury (33%). All patients in groups 1 and 2 were treated conservatively. A patient initially categorized in group 2, who had presented 5 months after injury, received surgical treatment

after conservative treatment failure. All patients in group 3 were also initially treated conservatively, but 9 received surgical treatment at a later stage because of instability. All group 4 patients underwent surgery and proceeded to have uneventful successful outcomes.

Differential Diagnosis

Suspected acute UCL injuries need to be discerned from diffuse capsular injury without discrete ligament tear, fracture or avulsions with

Table 1
Classification of UCL injury based on ligament appearance on MR imaging

Group	UCL Appearance	Treatment
1	Partial/undisplaced tear	Immobilization
2	Complete tear 3-mm displacement	Immobilization
3	Complete tear 3-mm displacement (buckled/quasi-Stener lesion)	Surgical repair
4	Stener lesion	Surgical repair

Recommended treatment based on MR imaging appearance as reported by Milner and colleagues.
From Milner CS, Manon-Matos Y, Thirkannad SM. Gamekeeper's thumb—a treatment-oriented magnetic resonance imaging classification. J Hand Surg Am 2015;40(1):90–5; with permission.

articular cartilage involvement, and arthritis. In chronic conditions, the degree of joint arthrosis needs to be determined, as this will guide treatment from a ligament reconstruction to MCP joint arthrodesis if the joint is arthritic.

On MR imaging, partial-thickness tears can be seen as thickening and abnormal signal of the ligament, often with focal defects within the substance of the ligament. Full-thickness tears of the collateral ligaments can be seen with complete discontinuity of the ligament and associated retraction or displacement of torn fibers. A Stener lesion is recognized by the displacement of the UCL with the adductor aponeurosis lying between the ligament and the underlying MCP joint. MRA demonstrates contrast extension from the joint through the torn ligament. MR imaging is also useful to determine if the UCL is torn off an avulsion fracture, as this finding may lead to operative intervention.

Treatment

Acute partial UCL injuries can be successfully treated nonoperatively. Acute, complete, or displaced UCL injuries as well as chronic injuries can be successfully treated with various operative strategies (see **Table 1**). If a painful arthrosis is present with chronic UCL instability, salvage may be performed with MCP joint fusion.[62]

ULNOTRIQUETRAL LIGAMENT TEAR
Anatomy

The UTL together with the ulnocapitate and the ulnolunate ligaments form the ulnocarpal complex. The TFCC attaches to the ulnar carpus via this complex. The UTL arises from the palmar radioulnar ligament and attaches to the palmar and ulnar triquetrum.[63]

Pathogenesis

Histologic sections demonstrate that the TFCC vasculature penetrates only the peripheral 10% to 40% leaving the central and radial portions of the TFCC avascular. Tears in hypovascular or avascular zones, therefore, tend to heal poorly. TFCC tears are subdivided into acute, traumatic, and chronic degenerative according to the Palmer classification.[64] Degeneration of the TFCC starts in the third decade of life so that by the fifth decade asymptomatic degenerative tears are common.[65] Traumatic injuries of the TFCC result from either the application of an extension, rotatory force to the axially loaded wrist, or a distraction force to the ulnar aspect of the wrist. Patients with isolated UTL split tears present with normal range of

motion.[66] Abnormal forearm rotation is suggestive of non-UTL pathology (eg, distal radioulnar joint (DRUJ) arthritis).[66] The ulnar fovea sign is a clinical maneuver reported to have a sensitivity and specificity of 90% and 88%, respectively, for UTL injury in the setting of a stable distal radioulnar joint, where the examiner places direct pressure over the UTL that lies distal and dorsal to the flexor carpi ulnaris tendon.[67] If the DRUJ is found to be unstable, foveal avulsion of the TFCC should be suspected.[66]

Imaging

The diagnostic workup should include plain radiographs and a neutral rotation posteroanterior and lateral view in order to assess for fractures, carpal malalignment, and ulnar variance. Radiographic examination of the DRUJ is concentrated to look for subluxation, arthritis, or ulnar styloid abnormalities.

Although central and radial TFCC tears have been shown to allow for reliable imaging on MR imaging,[39,68,69] peripheral sided TFCC tears can be more difficult to diagnose.[70,71] MR imaging can adequately diagnose complete, transverse UTL tears and foveal disruption of the TFCC with up to 100% sensitivity and specificity[68,72] (**Figs. 13** and **14**). However, longitudinal tears may present with more subtle imaging features and subsequently sensitivity ranges between 30% and 58%, with 60% specificity.[73] Longitudinal tears often have a smaller width than the resolution of the MR scanner and can, thus, also be hard to visualize.

During arthroscopy, tears in the UTL typically present with concomitant synovitis, a split of variable length, and intrasubstance perforations.[63,66]

Differential Diagnosis

Suspected UTL tears need to be differentiated from extensor carpi ulnaris subluxation, ulnar extrinsic ligament tear, DRUJ instability, pisotriquetral arthritis, ulnar artery thrombosis, ulnar neuropathy at the canal of Guyon, and dorsal ulnar sensory neuritis. At present, wrist arthroscopy is the gold standard to confirm a diagnosis of longitudinal split tear of the UTL.

Treatment

Patients with UTL tears may be treated nonoperatively with an above-elbow cast that limits prosupination. Arthroscopic treatment of longitudinal splits of the UTL results in improvement in grip strength and allows up to 90% of patients to return to full activity.[66]

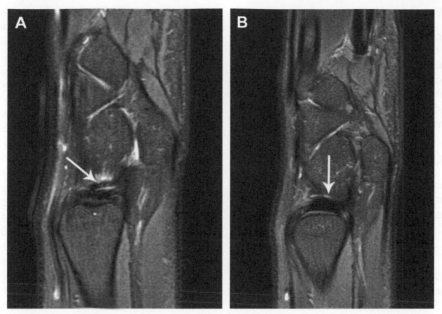

Fig. 13. Sagittal T2-weighted MR images with fat suppression going from ulnar (*A*) to radial (*B*) at the ulnar head. (*A*) There is a split tear of the UTL present extending longitudinally along the ligament with fluid interposed in the defect (*arrow*). (*B*) The slightly more radial image shows a normal disk of the TFCC (*arrow*).

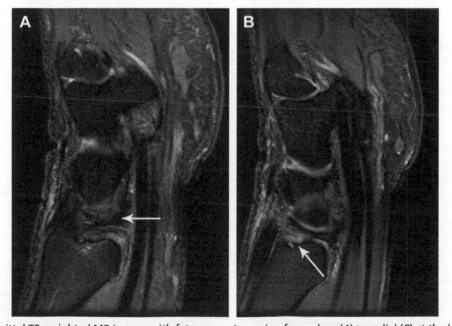

Fig. 14. Sagittal T2-weighted MR images with fat suppression going from ulnar (*A*) to radial (*B*) at the level of the ulnar head. (*A*) There is a high-grade tear of the UTL present (*arrow*). The UTL has lost its normal sharp margin and confluent low signal. (*B*) The tear extends through the disk of the TFCC and into the foveal attachment, which is completely torn from its attachment (*arrow*).

SUMMARY

The development of 3-T MR imaging scanners and dedicated wrist coils allows for new avenues of wrist imaging. They should be considered an extension of the physician's armamentarium as they can provide detailed anatomic examination of the unique anatomic structures within the hand and wrist which can guide treatment.

ACKNOWLEDGMENTS

The authors would like to thank Dr Kim Amrami, Department of Radiology at Mayo Clinic, for supplying some of the images within this article.

REFERENCES

1. Clark DC. Common acute hand infections. Am Fam Physician 2003;68:2167–76.
2. Schnall SB, Vu-Rose T, Holtom PD, et al. Tissue pressures in pyogenic flexor tenosynovitis of the finger. Compartment syndrome and its management. J Bone Joint Surg Br 1996;78:793–5.
3. DiFelice A, Seiler JG, Whitesides TE. The compartments of the hand: an anatomic study. J Hand Surg Am 1998;23:682–6.
4. Kanavel AB. Infections of the hand. Clin Orthop Relat Res 1974;104:3–8.
5. Siegel DB, Gelberman RH. Infections of the hand. Orthop Clin North Am 1988;19:779–89.
6. Ong YS, Levin LS. Hand infections. Plast Reconstr Surg 2009;124:225e–33e.
7. Gelberman RH, Menon J. The vascularity of the scaphoid bone. J Hand Surg Am 1980;5:508–13.
8. Slade JF, Dodds SD. Minimally invasive management of scaphoid nonunions. Clin Orthop Relat Res 2006;445:108–19.
9. Adams JE, Steinmann SP. Acute scaphoid fractures. Orthop Clin North Am 2007;38:229–35, vi.
10. Garcia RM, Ruch DS. Management of scaphoid fractures in the athlete: open and percutaneous fixation. Sports Med Arthrosc 2014;22:22–8.
11. Murthy NS. The role of magnetic resonance imaging in scaphoid fractures. J Hand Surg Am 2013;38:2047–54.
12. Waizenegger M, Barton NJ, Davis TR, et al. Clinical signs in scaphoid fractures. J Hand Surg Br 1994;19:743–7.
13. Hunter JC, Escobedo EM, Wilson AJ, et al. MR imaging of clinically suspected scaphoid fractures. AJR Am J Roentgenol 1997;168:1287–93.
14. Kusano N, Churei Y, Shiraishi E, et al. Diagnosis of occult carpal scaphoid fracture: a comparison of magnetic resonance imaging and computed tomography techniques. Tech Hand Up Extrem Surg 2002;6:119–23.
15. Brydie A, Raby N. Early MRI in the management of clinical scaphoid fracture. Br J Radiol 2003;76:296–300.
16. Patel NK, Davies N, Mirza Z, et al. Cost and clinical effectiveness of MRI in occult scaphoid fractures: a randomised controlled trial. Emerg Med J 2013;30:202–7.
17. Kirkeby L, Kairelyte V, Hansen TB. Early magnetic resonance imaging in patients with a clinically suspected scaphoid fracture may identify occult wrist injuries. J Hand Surg Eur Vol 2013;38:571–2.
18. Dorsay TA, Major NM, Helms CA. Cost-effectiveness of immediate MR imaging versus traditional follow-up for revealing radiographically occult scaphoid fractures. AJR Am J Roentgenol 2001;177:1257–63.
19. Cerezal L, Abascal F, Canga A, et al. Usefulness of gadolinium-enhanced MR imaging in the evaluation of the vascularity of scaphoid nonunions. AJR Am J Roentgenol 2000;174:141–9.
20. Schmitt R, Christopoulos G, Wagner M, et al. Avascular necrosis (AVN) of the proximal fragment in scaphoid nonunion: is intravenous contrast·agent necessary in MRI? Eur J Radiol 2011;77:222–7.
21. Fox MG, Gaskin CM, Chhabra AB, et al. Assessment of scaphoid viability with MRI: a reassessment of findings on unenhanced MR images. AJR Am J Roentgenol 2010;195:W281–6.
22. Sakai T, Sugano N, Nishii T, et al. MR findings of necrotic lesions and the extralesional area of osteonecrosis of the femoral head. Skeletal Radiol 2000;29:133–41.
23. Sebag G, Ducou Le Pointe H, Klein I, et al. Dynamic gadolinium-enhanced subtraction MR imaging–a simple technique for the early diagnosis of Legg-Calvé-Perthes disease: preliminary results. Pediatr Radiol 1997;27:216–20.
24. Cooney WP, Dobyns JH, Linscheid RL. Nonunion of the scaphoid: analysis of the results from bone grafting. J Hand Surg Am 1980;5:343–54.
25. Inoue G, Shionoya K, Kuwahata Y. Herbert screw fixation for scaphoid nonunions. An analysis of factors influencing outcome. Clin Orthop Relat Res 1997;(343):99–106.
26. Buijze GA, Goslings JC, Rhemrev SJ, et al. Cast immobilization with and without immobilization of the thumb for nondisplaced and minimally displaced scaphoid waist fractures: a multicenter, randomized, controlled trial. J Hand Surg Am 2014;39:621–7.
27. Majeed H. Non-operative treatment versus percutaneous fixation for minimally displaced scaphoid waist fractures in high demand young manual workers. J Orthop Traumatol 2014;15:239–44.
28. Dias JJ, Taylor M, Thompson J, et al. Radiographic signs of union of scaphoid fractures. An analysis of inter-observer agreement and reproducibility. J Bone Joint Surg Br 1988;70:299–301.

29. Kulkarni RW, Wollstein R, Tayar R, et al. Patterns of healing of scaphoid fractures. The importance of vascularity. J Bone Joint Surg Br 1999;81:85–90.

30. Imaeda T, Nakamura R, Miura T, et al. Magnetic resonance imaging in scaphoid fractures. J Hand Surg Br 1992;17:20–7.

31. McNally EG, Goodman R, Burge P. The role of MRI in the assessment of scaphoid fracture healing: a pilot study. Eur Radiol 2000;10:1926–8.

32. Dailiana ZH, Zachos V, Varitimidis S, et al. Scaphoid nonunions treated with vascularised bone grafts: MRI assessment. Eur J Radiol 2004;50:217–24.

33. Ganapathi M, Joseph G, Savage R, et al. MRI susceptibility artefacts related to scaphoid screws: the effect of screw type, screw orientation and imaging parameters. J Hand Surg Br 2002;27: 165–70.

34. Berger RA. The gross and histologic anatomy of the scapholunate interosseous ligament. J Hand Surg Am 1996;21:170–8.

35. Mayfield JK, Johnson RP, Kilcoyne RK. Carpal dislocations: pathomechanics and progressive perilunar instability. J Hand Surg Am 1980;5:226–41.

36. Ruch DS, Smith BP. Arthroscopic and open management of dynamic scaphoid instability. Orthop Clin North Am 2001;32:233–40, vii.

37. Gilula L, Mann F, Dobyns J, et al. Wrist terminology as defined by the international wrist investigators' workshop. J Bone Joint Surg 2002;1–66.

38. Linscheid RL, Dobyns JH, Beabout JW, et al. Traumatic instability of the wrist. Diagnosis, classification, and pathomechanics. J Bone Joint Surg Am 1972;54:1612–32.

39. Magee T. Comparison of 3-T MRI and arthroscopy of intrinsic wrist ligament and TFCC tears. AJR Am J Roentgenol 2009;192:80–5.

40. Walsh JJ, Berger RA, Cooney WP. Current status of scapholunate interosseous ligament injuries. J Am Acad Orthop Surg 2002;10:32–42.

41. Ringler MD. MRI of wrist ligaments. J Hand Surg Am 2013;38(10):2034–46.

42. Chim H, Moran SL. Wrist essentials: the diagnosis and management of scapholunate ligament injuries. Plast Reconstr Surg 2014;134:312e–22e.

43. Zlatkin MB, Chao PC, Osterman AL, et al. Chronic wrist pain: evaluation with high-resolution MR imaging. Radiology 1989;173:723–9.

44. Zlatkin MB, Rosner J. MR imaging of ligaments and triangular fibrocartilage complex of the wrist. Radiol Clin North Am 2006;44:595–623, ix.

45. Ruston J, Konan S, Rubinraut E, et al. Diagnostic accuracy of clinical examination and magnetic resonance imaging for common articular wrist pathology. Acta Orthop Belg 2013;79:375–80.

46. Bilateral arthrography of the wrist. 1990. Available at: http://www.sciencedirect.com/science/article/pii/026676819090129R.

47. Cantor RM, Stern PJ, Wyrick JD, et al. The relevance of ligament tears or perforations in the diagnosis of wrist pain: an arthrographic study. J Hand Surg Am 1994;19:945–53.

48. Theumann NH, Etechami G, Duvoisin B, et al. Association between extrinsic and intrinsic carpal ligament injuries at MR arthrography and carpal instability at radiography: initial observations. Radiology 2006;238:950–7.

49. Lee YH, Choi YR, Kim S, et al. Intrinsic ligament and triangular fibrocartilage complex (TFCC) tears of the wrist: comparison of isovolumetric 3D-THRIVE sequence MR arthrography and conventional MR image at 3 T. Magn Reson Imaging 2013;31:221–6.

50. Garcia-Elias M, Lluch AL, Stanley JK. Three-ligament tenodesis for the treatment of scapholunate dissociation: indications and surgical technique. J Hand Surg Am 2006;31:125–34.

51. Stener B. Displacement of the ruptured ulnar collateral ligament of the metacarpo-phalangeal joint of the thumb: a clinical and anatomical study. J Bone Joint Surg Br 1962;11:869–79.

52. Smith RJ. Post-traumatic instability of the metacarpophalangeal joint of the thumb. J Bone Joint Surg Am 1977;59:14–21.

53. Campbell C. 'Gamekeeper's thumb. J Bone Joint Surg Br 1955;37:148–9.

54. Heyman P, Gelberman RH, Duncan K, et al. Injuries of the ulnar collateral ligament of the thumb metacarpophalangeal joint. Biomechanical and prospective clinical studies on the usefulness of valgus stress testing. Clin Orthop Relat Res 1993;(292): 165–71.

55. Malik AK, Morris T, Chou D, et al. Clinical testing of ulnar collateral ligament injuries of the thumb. J Hand Surg Eur Vol 2009;34:363–6.

56. Harper MT, Chandnani VP, Spaeth J, et al. Gamekeeper thumb: diagnosis of ulnar collateral ligament injury using magnetic resonance imaging, magnetic resonance arthrography and stress radiography. J Magn Reson Imaging 1996;6:322–8.

57. Hergan K, Mittler C. Sonography of the injured ulnar collateral ligament of the thumb. J Bone Joint Surg Br 1995;77:77–83.

58. Susic D, Hansen BR, Hansen TB. Ultrasonography may be misleading in the diagnosis of ruptured and dislocated ulnar collateral ligaments of the thumb. Scand J Plast Reconstr Surg Hand Surg 1999;33:319–20.

59. Hergan K, Mittler C, Oser W. Ulnar collateral ligament: differentiation of displaced and nondisplaced tears with US and MR imaging. Radiology 1995;194:65–71.

60. Romano WM, Garvin G, Bhayana D, et al. The spectrum of ulnar collateral ligament injuries as viewed on magnetic resonance imaging of the metacarpophalangeal joint of the thumb. Can Assoc Radiol J 2003;54:243–8.

61. Milner CS, Manon-Matos Y, Thirkannad SM. Game-keeper's thumb—a treatment-oriented magnetic resonance imaging classification. J Hand Surg Am 2015;40:90–5.

62. Rhee PC, Jones DB, Kakar S. Management of thumb metacarpophalangeal ulnar collateral ligament injuries. J Bone Joint Surg Am 2012;94:2005–12.

63. Berger RA. The anatomy of the ligaments of the wrist and distal radioulnar joints. Clin Orthop Relat Res 2001;(383):32–40.

64. Palmer AK. Triangular fibrocartilage complex lesions: a classification. J Hand Surg Am 1989;14:594–606.

65. Mikić ZD. Age changes in the triangular fibrocartilage of the wrist joint. J Anat 1978;126:367–84.

66. Tay SC, Berger RA, Parker WL. Longitudinal split tears of the ulnotriquetral ligament. Hand Clin 2010;26:495–501.

67. Tay SC, Tomita K, Berger RA. The 'ulnar fovea sign' for defining ulnar wrist pain: an analysis of sensitivity and specificity. J Hand Surg Am 2007;32:438–44.

68. Anderson ML, Skinner JA, Felmlee JP, et al. Diagnostic comparison of 1.5 tesla and 3.0 tesla preoperative MRI of the wrist in patients with ulnar-sided wrist pain. J Hand Surg Am 2008; 33:1153–9.

69. Hobby JL, Tom BD, Bearcroft PW, et al. Magnetic resonance imaging of the wrist: diagnostic performance statistics. Clin Radiol 2001;56:50–7.

70. Haims AH, Schweitzer ME, Morrison WB, et al. Limitations of MR imaging in the diagnosis of peripheral tears of the triangular fibrocartilage of the wrist. AJR Am J Roentgenol 2002;178:419–22.

71. Zanetti M, Linkous MD, Gilula LA, et al. Characteristics of triangular fibrocartilage defects in symptomatic and contralateral asymptomatic wrists. Radiology 2000;216:840–5.

72. Totterman SM, Miller RJ, McCance SE, et al. Lesions of the triangular fibrocartilage complex: MR findings with a three-dimensional gradient-recalled-echo sequence. Radiology 1996;199:227–32.

73. Ringler MD, Howe BM, Amrami KK, et al. Utility of magnetic resonance imaging for detection of longitudinal split tear of the ulnotriquetral ligament. J Hand Surg Am 2013;38:1723–7.

Index

Note: Page numbers of article titles are in **boldface** type.

Magn Reson Imaging Clin N Am 23 (2015) 511–514
http://dx.doi.org/10.1016/S1064-9689(15)00071-9
1064-9689/15/$ – see front matter © 2015 Elsevier Inc. All rights reserved.

mri.theclinics.com

Moving?

Make sure your subscription moves with you!

To notify us of your new address, find your **Clinics Account Number** (located on your mailing label above your name), and contact customer service at:

Email: journalscustomerservice-usa@elsevier.com

800-654-2452 (subscribers in the U.S. & Canada)
314-447-8871 (subscribers outside of the U.S. & Canada)

Fax number: 314-447-8029

Elsevier Health Sciences Division
Subscription Customer Service
3251 Riverport Lane
Maryland Heights, MO 63043

*To ensure uninterrupted delivery of your subscription,
please notify us at least 4 weeks in advance of move.

Printed and bound by CPI Group (UK) Ltd, Croydon, CR0 4YY

03/10/2024

01040378-0017